Telepractice in Audiology

Editor-in-Chief for Audiology

Brad A. Stach, PhD

Telepractice in Audiology

Emma Rushbrooke, MPhil(AUD), BA, DipAud.,
MAudA., LSLS. Cert. AVT, RNC

K. Todd Houston, PhD, CCC-SLP, LSLS Cert. AVT

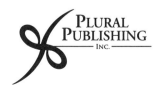

PLURAL
PUBLISHING
INC.

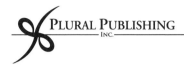

5521 Ruffin Road
San Diego, CA 92123

e-mail: info@pluralpublishing.com
Website: http://www.pluralpublishing.com

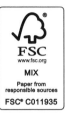

Typeset in 11/13 Garamond Book by Flanagan's Publishing Services, Inc.
Printed in the United States of America by McNaughton & Gunn, Inc.

Library of Congress Cataloging-in-Publication Data

Telepractice in audiology / [edited by] Emma Rushbrooke, K. Todd Houston.
    p. ; cm.
  Includes bibliographical references and index.
  ISBN 978-1-59756-613-1 (alk. paper)—ISBN 1-59756-613-6 (alk. paper)
  I. Rushbrooke, Emma, editor. II. Houston, K. Todd, editor.
  [DNLM: 1. Audiology. 2. Diffusion of Innovation. 3. Hearing Disorders.
4. Telemedicine. WV 270]
  RF290
  617.8—dc23
                                                          2015026489

Contents

Foreword

The emergence of telepractice in audiology represents a major change in audiological practice; in fact, it is the single biggest change that I have observed in my 35-year professional career. Telepractice has the potential to radically alter existing service delivery systems, to provide audiology services to millions who would otherwise not have benefited from them, and, importantly, to improve the level of re/habilitation for people with hearing loss around the world.

Although extremely important for developing countries that are underserved by professional services and for countries like Australia where the tyranny of distance means that professional services do not reach all those in need, its application is not limited to such environments. Adults and children living in urban areas in developed countries can also benefit from rapid, easy access to high-quality audiological support.

Thus, the emergence of this first book on *Telepractice in Audiology* is incredibly timely. I do understand, however, that change can be threatening in many ways, and there are consumers, clinicians, researchers, and policy makers who are concerned about the new practice and how it will work for them. I would encourage all to heed the words of Mahatma Gandhi, who encouraged us to become actively involved in change; he said, "Be the change that you wish to see in the world."

The first change management step in adopting a new mode of practice is to gain knowledge about the new practice, and this book is an outstanding source of information for that knowledge. It brings together details about the history of telepractice in audiology; existing telepractice in diagnosis, hearing aid fitting, cochlear implant mapping, and re/habilitation; methods of evaluating the outcomes of telepractice in audiology; and the potential for future telepractice applications.

The book is edited by clinicians/researchers with extensive expertise in this field: Emma Rushbrooke and Todd Houston. I have known Emma since she first studied audiology at the University of Queensland and, in recent years, I supervised her excellent research master's study that evaluated the validity of remote cochlear implant mapping for children. Both Emma and Todd are committed to developing the evidence base needed to underpin telepractice in audiology, and in this book, they have gathered together an outstanding team of contributing authors to provide that evidence.

Finally, I recommend this book to consumers, clinicians, researchers, and policy makers—the change to telepractice in audiology is upon us, and reading this book will help us all to be a part of that change.

> —Louise Hickson, BSpThy(Hons), MAud, PhD
> Head, School of Health and Rehabilitation
>   Sciences
> Professor of Audiology, Co-Director,
>   Communication Disability Centre
> The University of Queensland, Australia

Acknowledgments

The process of creating a new book is challenging but, instilled in the process, is the shared focus of so many talented individuals. We have thoroughly enjoyed the opportunities to collaborate and learn from all who lent their time and expertise to ensure that we produced an excellent book on the topic of *Telepractice in Audiology*.

To that end, we wish to extend our deepest appreciation to our international cast of contributing authors who so generously gave their time and shared their knowledge and experience in the area of telepractice. We believe that many will benefit from your insights and will be inspired to incorporate telepractice into their service provision.

We also would like to sincerely thank the editors and staff at Plural Publishing, especially Valerie Johns, Rachel Singer, Megan Carter, Kalie Koscielak, and Alya Hameed for their guidance and support from the development of the initial concept of the book through the writing, editing, and production processes. We appreciated your encouragement, patience, and consistent professionalism.

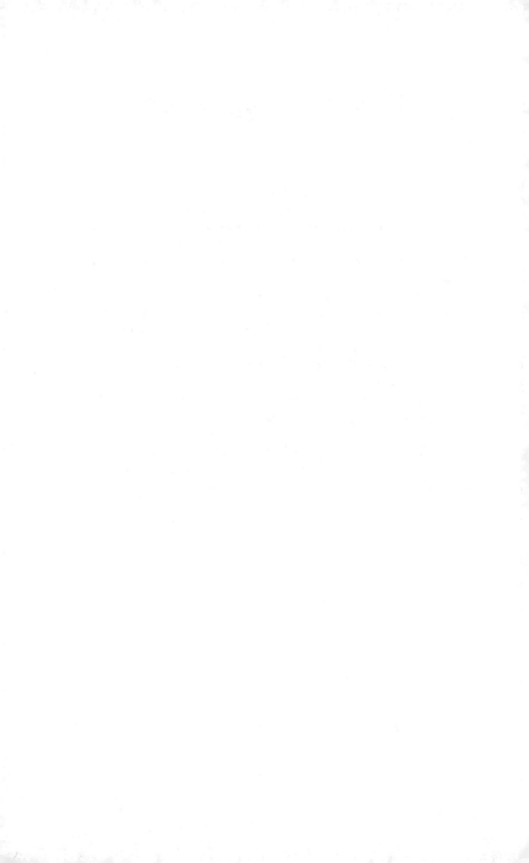

Contributors

Beth Atkinson, BSpPath, MAudSt, MAudA (CCP)
Clinical Manager
Audiology
Hear and Say
Brisbane, Australia
Chapter 8

Jackie Brown, BEd (Deafness Studies), DipTeach, LSLS Cert. AVT
Education and Development Manager
Hear and Say
Brisbane, Australia
Chapter 9

Gabriella Constantinescu, PhD, BSpPath (Hons)
Lecturer in Speech Pathology
School of Allied and Public Health
Faculty of Health Sciences
Australian Catholic University
Melbourne, Australia
Chapter 10

Dimity Dornan, AO, PhD UQ, HonDUniv USQ, BSpThy, FSPAA, CpSp, LSLS Cert. AVT
Executive Director and Founder
Hear and Say
Associate Professor
University of Queensland
Associate Professor
Griffith University
Brisbane, Australia
Chapter 10

Robert H. Eikelboom, BEng, MApplSc, PhD
Adjunct Associate Professor
Ear Sciences Centre, School of Surgery
The University of Western Australia
Nedlands, Australia

Head eHealth Group
Ear Science Institute Australia
Subiaco, Australia
Extra-ordinary Professor
Department of Speech-Language Pathology and Audiology
University of Pretoria
Pretoria, South Africa
Chapters 5 and 11

Carolyn Evans, BSc, MAud, MAudA (CCP)
Audiologist
Hear and Say
Brisbane, Australia
Chapter 9

David A. Fabry, PhD
Vice President
Audiology and Professional Relations
Starkey Hearing Technologies
Minneapolis, Minnesota
Chapter 6

Lynda Farwell, BSpPath, LSLS Cert. AVT
Team Leader–Listening and Spoken Language
Hear and Say
Brisbane, Australia
Chapter 7

Catherine M. McMahon, PhD
Associate Professor
Head of Audiology
Department of Linguistics
Macquarie University
Sydney, Australia
Chapter 3

K. Todd Houston, PhD, CCC-SLP, LSLS Cert. AVT
Professor
School of Speech-Language Pathology and Audiology
College of Health Professions
The University of Akron
Akron, OH

Chapters 1 and 7

Colleen Psarros, BAppSc (SpPath), MSc(AUD), MAudA(CCP)
Clinical Practice and Strategy Manager
SCIC (an RIDBC service)
Gladesville, Sydney, Australia
Chapters 3 and 4

Emma Rushbrooke, MPhil(AUD), BA, DipAud., MAudA., LSLS Cert. AVT, RNC
Clinical Director
Hear and Say
Brisbane, Australia
Chapters 1, 2, and 8

Michelle von Muralt, BSpPath, LSLS Cert AVT
Team Leader–Listening and Spoken Language
Hear and Say
Brisbane, Australia
Chapter 7

De Wet Swanepoel, PhD
Professor
Department of Speech-Language Pathology and Audiology
University of Pretoria
Pretoria, South Africa
Adjunct Associate Professor
Ear Sciences Centre, School of Surgery
The University of Western Australia
Nedlands, Australia
Senior Research Fellow
Ear Science Institute Australia
Subiaco, Australia
Chapters 5 and 11

Emma van Wanrooy, BA, MAud, MAudA (CCP)
Audiologist
(Formerly at SCIC)
Pittwater Hearing
Avalon, Sydney, Australia
Chapter 4

*This book is dedicated to all the children and families
who benefit from Telepractice, and to my work colleagues
whose passion and innovation constantly inspire me.
Deep appreciation goes to my wonderful husband Darren,
family and friends, whose unfailing understanding,
encouragement and support have made this work possible.
Lastly, to my ever faithful Milo, who waited patiently for walks
and kept me company throughout—no matter what the time!*

—Emma Rushbrooke

*Like Emma, I'd like to dedicate this book to all of the children,
families, and adults with hearing loss who continue to
teach me so much about telepractice. I will remain eternally
grateful for your patience and support as we work together
to forge new ways of delivering vital services at a distance.*

*I also have to thank my colleagues on faculty in the School of
Speech-Language Pathology and Audiology at the University
of Akron for your willingness to tolerate my clinical and
research interests in telepractice and hearing loss. As well,
I must thank the dedicated graduate students in speech-
language pathology that I have the honor and privilege
to work beside every day. You continue to inspire me.*

*And finally, I'd like to thank my wife, Maria, for tolerating the
long hours, distracted conversations, and my need to sit in
front of my computer for extended periods of time. Thank you
for being my partner in all of the things that matter in life.*

—K. Todd Houston

1

History, Terminology, and the Advent of Teleaudiology

Emma Rushbrooke and K. Todd Houston

Key Points

- Technology is a tool that enables innovation.
- Reviewing the past helps us to better understand the impact of innovation.
- The dynamic nature of this field has led to evolving terminology, descriptions, applications, and service delivery models.
- Telehealth is an umbrella term, and teleaudiology is an application of telecommunication technology to provide a range of diagnostic and treatment services to individuals with hearing loss.

Recent advances in technology have made communication and information access faster, less expensive, and more accessible than ever. These technologies afford a tremendous opportunity to grow telepractice and redefine where, when, and how care is provided. Looking back at the history of telepractice yields important lessons and provides guidance for how we can move forward, most significantly, as it relates to the role of technology as an enabling infrastructure. (Brennan, 2013, p. 4)

For more than a century, physicians, clinicians, and other health care providers have been investigating the use of information and communication technology to improve access to health care. Continued innovation and advances have enabled the development of many types of *tele*communication systems and, by extension, potential models of service delivery. The ability that clinicians now have to use real-time audio and video transmission, faster broadband Internet access, reduced costs, increased portability, and the rapid diffusion of wireless mobile devices means that this type of service provision is more accessible than ever before (Armstrong, Giovinco, Joseph, Mills, & Rogers, 2011; Dzenowagis, 2009; Houston, 2014; Houston, Fleming, Brown, Weinberg, & Nafe, 2014; Xiaohui et al., 2013). Information and communication technologies are widely viewed as having great potential to transform the delivery of health care on a global scale. However, although these technological advances have provided many opportunities, it is important to emphasize that the technology is just a tool (Brennan, 2013; Cohn, 2013), and it will be the innovations of the practitioners using this technology that will enable the true integration of telecommunication or telepractice into hearing health care.

Reports and documentation relating to the use of distance communication to relay messages about significant events or medical or health information, date back over many centuries (Field, 1996; Houston et al., 2014; Zundel, 1996). From visual and sound signals such as bonfires, horns, and drums to the present-day use of the Internet, humans have found innovative methods of communication to relay information over great distances (Constantinescu, 2010; Houston et al., 2014). As noted above, technological advancement has resulted in what is now referred to as forms of "tele" communication. The prefix *tele* is the Greek root word for *distant* or *remote* (Darkins & Cary, 2000; Houston et al., 2014) and, as such, defines information and communication delivery over a distance.

The use of information and communication technology in the delivery of medical or health-related services (telehealth) is growing and changing, and new applications are emerging. The area of telehealth is not a single entity or discipline but instead a number of different and evolving applications. The rapid adoption of telehealth models across a range of disciplines has resulted in changing terminology being used to describe and define these different applications. Although this is representative of a dynamic model of service provision, some of the literature suggests that this has led to a lack of clarity and some disagreement about definitions and concepts (Bashshur, Shannon, Krupinski, & Grigsby, 2011; Fatehi & Wootton, 2012; Wootton, Patil, Scott, & Ho, 2009).

This chapter provides an overview of the history of telehealth and more specifically, telepractice in audiology (i.e., teleaudiology). The terminology associated with this field also is discussed and explored. The authors believe that looking back to the past and the evolution that has occurred to the present day allows us to better understand the impact of innovation and the future potential of telepractice intervention (Brennan, 2013; Houston & Behl, 2012).

Overview of the History

The idea of using communication devices to transmit health care or medical information is not new; however, it is an area that has evolved due to technological advancement, necessity, and demand (Constantinescu, 2010; Darkins & Cary, 2000). Although there is some disagreement in the literature as to the exact origins of distance communication (Houston et al., 2014), what is important is that there is a long history that highlights the impact of distance on access and the importance of connectivity within and between societies (Bashshur & Shannon, 2009). Throughout time, humans have used their own bodies and available "technologies"—even if they were rather primitive compared to today's standards—to manage the tyranny of distance. In antiquity, for example, messengers would run between villages and city-states to share the critical news of the day. By the Middle Ages, the use of bonfires and flags to relay medical information about the bubonic plague was one of the earliest means of distance health communication (Constantinescu, 2010; Craig & Patterson, 2006; Darkins & Cary, 2000; Zundel, 1996).

From Postal Systems to the Telephone

Although not very reliable, postal systems were used in the 1700s by physicians for health-related management and diagnosis (Constantinescu, 2010; Craig & Patterson, 2006; Darkins & Cary, 2000; Houston et al., 2010; Zundel, 1996). The early 19th century saw the use of the modern heliograph and the telegraph. The heliograph is a mirror system that reflects sunlight. When manipulated in specific ways, the reflected sunlight can produce coded messages. The first recorded use of a primitive heliograph was in 405 BCE when the ancient Greeks used polished shields to send messages in battle. The modern heliograph design, which incorporates a tripod and adjustable frame, is attributed to Carl Friedrich Gauss (Bashshur & Shannon, 2009) and was used in the 1800s to signal information about death rates resulting from war or famine (Houston et al., 2010; Zundel, 1996).

A more reliable technology, the telegraph, was invented in the mid-1800s by Samuel Morse (Constantinescu, 2010; Craig & Patterson, 2006; Darkins & Cary, 2000; Houston et al., 2010; Zundel, 1996). Morse, a highly respected artist and portrait painter at the time, was motivated to develop the telegraph after experiencing the unexpected death of his wife. While away in Washington, D.C., completing a commissioned painting, he received word via horse messenger that his wife was having a very difficult pregnancy and had become quite ill. He immediately returned to his home in New Haven, Connecticut, but he arrived too late. His wife had died and was buried (Houston et al., 2010). Feeling deep sadness and remorse for the loss of his beloved wife, Morse abandoned painting and devoted the rest of his life to developing the telegraph.

By 1844, Morse had secured the funding to develop the telegraph, and he tested his new invention by sending a message from the U.S. Capitol building to a site in Baltimore, Maryland. Using a code (i.e., Morse code) that he and his colleagues had developed, Morse's first message was, "What hath God wrought." News of this new invention quickly spread, and within a decade, telegraph lines and transmitter stations populated cities and communities on the East Coast, in the Midwest, and in the South. The telegraph and the growing dominance of the railroad for mass transportation and shipping are credited as important factors in the westward expansion of the United States (Dilts, 1996). For ease and convenience, telegraph lines often were installed along railroad tracks.

During the American Civil War (1861–1865), the telegraph was used extensively to issue commands to troops on both sides of the conflict and to report troop movements. More importantly, it was also used to report casualty lists and to secure scarce medical supplies. Although the telegraph proved to be an important technological step in the communication of medical information, it also is critical to note that Morse code has outlived the device. Various first responders, militaries, and other civil service personnel continue to use the code to relay information in situations when other devices are nonfunctional.

While Morse perfected wired communication, a relatively unknown inventor, Mahlon Loomis, experimented with what he called "wireless telegraphy" (Huurdeman, 2003). In 1866, he demonstrated his invention between two mountain peaks in Virginia. Although mostly lost to history, Loomis' invention was a forerunner to the radio, but it would be another 30 years before the Italian inventor, Guglielmo Marconi, would be credited with its invention in 1895.

Later in the 19th century, one of the most significant inventions in history, the telephone, was invented by Dr. Alexander Graham Bell, a noted inventor, scientist, and teacher of the deaf. Dr. Bell's patent in 1876 described this new device as his "Improvements of Telegraphy." Although other inventors, such as Philipp Reis, Elisha Gray, and Antonio Meucci, had developed similar devices, it was Bell who perfected the magnetic microphone, which made the telephone commercially feasible (Chakravorty, 1976). Interestingly, it was an incident in 1875 involving Dr. Bell and his lab assistant, Thomas Watson, that not only signaled the invention of a new communication device but could also possibly be the first documented example of someone seeking medical intervention using "modern" technology. Bell summoned his lab assistant to help him after spilling acid on his hand or leg (Carson, 2007).

Over time, Bell eventually realized the broad and far-reaching impact that the telephone had on mass communication. However, his early experiments focused on how to transmit sound, especially speech, across a wire. Bell, a noted elocutionist (i.e., a speech-language pathologist of his day) and teacher of the deaf, knew that if he could manipulate speech and make it louder, such a device could be a tremendous aid in teaching children with hearing loss how to listen and acquire spoken language.

Bell became quite famous for the invention of the telephone; however, he believed that his photophone would be recognized as his greatest and most important invention (Carson, 2007). The photophone was designed to use a modulated light beam to transmit a person's voice over a distance. Both the transmitter and receiver consisted of a plane of mirrors and a selenium cell. The modulating light from the transmitter would be interpreted as a speech signal and would be reproduced in the receiver. The first wireless telephone message was transmitted by Bell through the photophone in Washington, D.C., in April 1880.

Unfortunately, Bell's wish for the photophone to revolutionize telephone communication would not be immediately realized. Because the photophone depended on bright light for signal transmission, he could not overcome the effects of inclement weather. However, the basic concepts employed by the photophone became the precursors for modern fiber-optic communication, which uses light to transmit large amounts of information at extremely high speeds.

Although Bell will be remembered as the inventor of the telephone, his professional and scientific interests varied widely. He made significant contributions to the study of the genetics of deafness, home air conditioning, vertical flight with the help of rotors (forerunner to today's helicopters), heavier-than-air flying machines (i.e., airplanes), hydrofoil boats, artificial ventilation for underwater breathing, and a device to detect foreign metal objects (i.e., a metal detector), such as a bullet, in human tissue (Chakravorty, 1976). And finally, Bell's connection with deafness and audiology was both personal and professional. His mother, Eliza, was deaf, and he later married Mabel Hubbard, who also was deaf. He was intimately involved in the development of the audiometer, an instrument that could measure aural acuity but also permitted differentiation in the degrees of deafness. Bell's remedial teaching of spoken language could then be tailored to the individual's specific learning and communication needs (Chakravorty, 1976).

By the beginning of the 20th century, telephones were in widespread use, and physicians were among the early adopters of its use in medical care. Gunsch (2011) postulates that tele-medicine began—on a limited basis—in the early 1900s when electrocardiograms were transmitted over telephone lines, and physicians were able to read the test results. By 1910, telephones were used to transmit amplified stethoscope sounds as well as electroencephalograms (a graphic record of the electrical activity of the brain) (Constantinescu, 2010; Gunsch, 2011; Houston et al., 2010).

From Radio to the Birth of Modern Telepractice in Health Care

By the early 1900s, radio communication was being rapidly adopted as a new wireless means by which medical and health care services could be successfully provided at a distance. As a matter of convenience, physicians and other medical person-nel used radio to provide consultations to patients who were in more remote locations. By the 1920s, radio transmissions were being used by doctors to treat and counsel sailors during medical emergencies at sea. This form of communication was a valuable source of medical contact for seafarers and is still used extensively today in most militaries, by civil servants, and by first responders when emergencies occur (Constantinescu, 2010; Craig & Patterson, 2006; Houston & Behl, 2012). Interestingly, in the early 1900s in Australia, bicycle-powered radios were used by the Australian Royal Flying Doctors to communicate medical information across large distances (*Teleradiology*, n.d.).

The introduction of the television was a milestone in both entertainment and communication, and the television provided a new means of relaying medical or health care information. Constantinescu (2010) notes that that the birth of "modern" tele-health occurred with the introduction of both the television and satellite communication (Bashshur, Reardon, & Shannon, 2000; Constantinescu, 2010) in the 1950s. In terms of medical applica-tions, the ability to see a patient's condition rather than rely on an audio description greatly enhanced the diagnostic process as well as the confidence of those engaged in treatment (House & Roberts, 1977). Some of the first medical uses of television date back to 1959 in the United States (Bashshur & Shannon, 2009; Perednia & Allen, 1995). In that year, clinicians at the University of Nebraska used two-way, closed-circuit, interactive television to transmit information and neurological assessments across the university campus to medical students (Bashshur & Shannon, 2009). They next applied its use for group therapy consultations and, in 1964, used closed-circuit television to provide a direct communication between the Nebraska Psychiatric Institute in Omaha and the Norfolk State Mental Hospital. These institutions were separated by a distance of more than 100 miles (Bashshur & Shannon, 2009; Benschoter, Wittson, & Ingham, 1965; Constantinescu, 2010; Houston et al., 2014). The communication link allowed medical practitioners to successfully perform consultations and neurological examinations with patients and also facilitated training and education at a distance (Bashshur & Shannon, 2009; Constantinescu, 2010; Houston et al., 2014). Later, in the late 1960s and early 1970s, two-way interactive microwave communication technology was used between the Massachusetts General Hospital and Logan International Airport Medical Station in Boston. This service allowed for the delivery of 24/7 medical care to airport passengers and staff (Constantinescu, 2010; Houston et al., 2014; Murphy & Bird, 1974).

The space race started in the 1950s and was well under way by the 1960s. The pioneering efforts to develop and launch satellites had many beneficial outcomes with regard to information and communication technology. The National Aeronautics and Space Administration (NASA) was interested in monitoring the health of astronauts in space via satellite communication (Bashshur et al., 2000; Constantinescu, 2010; Craig & Patterson, 2006; Houston et al., 2014; Welsh, 1999; Zundel, 1996). NASA's success in the monitoring of astronauts using satellite technology assisted in the development of telehealth programs for rural and remote populations and also offered significant potential for disaster relief interventions (Constantinescu, 2010). In another project, NASA, in collaboration with Lockheed and the USA Public Health Service, initiated the Space Technology Applied to Rural Papago Advanced Health Care (STARPAHC) program. The program provided general medical services via satellite-based communications to the people of the Papago Indian Reservation in Arizona (Constantinescu, 2010; Fuchs, 1979; Houston et al., 2014; Maheu, Whitten, & Allen, 2001; Stanberry, 1998a). This program was active from 1973 to 1977, and is significant because it demonstrated the success and effectiveness of a telepractice model (Houston et al., 2014).

Satellite technology was next used for disaster relief and assisted with rescue operations across the world. An example is the 1985 Advanced Technology-3 satellite (ATS-3) that facilitated communication between the American Red Cross and the Pan American Health Organization in earthquake-stricken Mexico City (Constantinescu, 2010; Garshnek & Burkle, 1999a, 1999b). The ATS-3 enabled voice communication support for the international rescue and relief teams. This communication link was vital, as the earthquake had disabled the majority of land-based forms of communication in Mexico City (Garshnek & Burkle, 1999b).

The Department of Veterans Affairs (VA) in the United States also played a significant role in the advancement of telepractice in health care. The VA started using telemedicine in the 1970s to treat neurogenic communicative disorders, and it continues to innovate and use these services today in many areas of rehabilitation. Before this innovative care was introduced, veterans had to travel to the VA hospital or medical center for their health care needs. This was not always a viable option, as approximately 37% of veterans reside in rural areas (Dennis, Gladden, & Noe, 2012; Houston et al., 2014). In order to reduce long travel times and improve access for veterans, the VA established over 800 community-based outpatient clinics (CBOCs) to provide care closer to the patient's place of residence. Unfortunately, however, there was a shortage of trained staff and specialty services at these clinics. The VA recognized that this shortage meant that specialty health services were unavailable to the majority of those residing in rural areas. To assist in addressing this, the Office of Telehealth Services (OTS) was established in 2003, making available an array of health care services to improve access to health care and hopefully lead to better health outcomes. The OTS was established to support the development of new health care delivery models that use cutting-edge health information technologies. Following its establishment, the OTS began deploying its clinic-based telehealth in the areas of telemental health in 2003, telerehabilitation in 2005, teleretinal imaging also in 2005, and primary care telehealth in 2011. The VA has continued to innovate in telepractice, resulting in three main areas of focus: Clinical Video Telehealth (CVT), Home Telehealth (HT), and Store and Forward Telehealth (SFT). As of 2012, around 600,000 veterans were receiving services through telepractice (Dennis et al., 2012; Houston et al., 2014).

The success of the initiatives discussed above highlights the potential and effectiveness of the telepractice model of service delivery. However, despite these promising outcomes, the great majority of projects initiated prior to 1986 were not sustainable. This was in large part due to high costs, the quality of the technology available at the time, and the lack of sustained government funding (Bashshur et al., 2000; Constaninescu, 2010; Houston et al., 2014; Maheu et al., 2001).

1990s Through to Today: Rebirth Driven by Technological Advancements

During the 1990s and 2000s, renewed interest in telepractice began to escalate. This resurgence was driven by advances in digital communication technology and the Internet. Reduced costs associated with the technology and infrastructure, as well as social influence and political pressure, also assisted in the push for more telehealth services (Constantinescu, 2010; Houston et al., 2014; Maheu et al., 2001; Whitten, Frances, & Collins, 1997). Constantinescu (2010) notes that there was increasing concern regarding the inequity of access to health care for rural and remote populations, and the rising costs of health care assisted in the push to investigate alternative models of service provision (Constantinescu, 2010).

The advances in digital communication technology enabled interactive desktop or network computer-based videoconferencing over lower bandwidth, and Internet connections were a much more cost-effective option to the more expensive satellite alternative (Constantinescu, 2010; Maheu et al., 2001). The reduced costs associated with computing technology (e.g., laptops, tablets, smartphones) and the increased availability of online software and teleconferencing websites (e.g., Skype, Google Talk, FaceTime) have made real-time videoconferencing much more accessible and even mobile (Houston, Behl, & Walters, 2013). In addition, the easier access and usability of videoconferencing and the increased speed and quality of data transfer have resulted in a heightened awareness and support of telehealth as a practical option for the delivery of medical and health-related services (Constantinescu, 2010; Kuo, Delvecchio, Babayan, & Preminger 2001; Mun & Turner, 1999).

Dzenowagis (2009) notes that the amazing growth in the diffusion of information and communication technology across the world has resulted in social and cultural changes, which have in turn facilitated the integration of this technology into everyday life. The consumers or stakeholders of this technology have had a significant impact on shaping this growth and integration into the mainstream, and there is a greater awareness of the positive impacts of improved access on a global scale. Of note, 2014 statistics show a 741% growth in world Internet usage in the past 14 years, and it has currently penetrated approximately 40% of the global population (International Telecommunications Union, 2014; Internet World Stats, 2014). By the end of 2014, there were almost 3 billion Internet users globally. Two thirds of these Internet users were from the developing world where the number of Internet users has doubled in the past 5 years, from 974 million to 1.9 billion (International Telecommunications Union, 2014).

Terminology

The overview of the history in this field has shown that the use of information and communication technology to deliver health services has grown and continues to evolve. Human innovation, together with new technologies, changing health needs, and "societal demographic pressure" (Craig & Miskelly, 2010, p. 1), has resulted in the emergence of many different technological applications. Although this is representative of a dynamic model of service provision, it has resulted in many new terms or definitions being used. Although the development of new terminology may help to distinguish emerging applications from historical ones, some of the literature suggests that the debate around terminology may be contributing to a lack of clarity and standardization in this area of health services provision (Bashshur et al., 2011; Craig & Miskelly, 2010; Fatehi & Wootton, 2012).

Kazely, McLeod, and Wager (2012) note that the lack of language commonality could be considered one of the barriers in this field. The interchangeability of terms may result in confusion for the clients or participants in the health service, and this can also lead to apprehension. The lack of consistency also means that there is no universal term being used by policy makers, government agencies, and other decision makers (Stredler-Brown, 2014). In addition, this confusion in terminology and classification may impact research, further development, and implementation. Most importantly, the terminology must be relevant to the client or consumer (Kamat, 2010). Thus, standardized definitions and terminology are important within this field in order to reduce misunderstandings and confusion experienced by key stakeholders, industry insiders, and consumers.

There are many different overarching or umbrella terms used to describe the provision of distance services using information and communication technology. Some of these include telemedicine, telehealth, telepractice, and eHealth (Givens & Elangovan, 2003; Krumm, 2007; Rushbrooke, 2012). Telemedicine generally relates more to the delivery of remote medical care or curative medicine, with this terminology first introduced in the 1970s. Telehealth emerged later, in the 1990s, and was supposed to be a more inclusive term to describe distant health care and extend the scope of service provision (Constantinescu, 2010; Craig & Patterson, 2006; Givens & Elangovan, 2003; Maheu et al., 2001; Stanberry, 1998a; van Dyk, 2014). More recently, around the year 2000, the term eHealth started to be used and includes aspects related to data management, clinical information, and processing in addition to patient services (Swanepoel, 2013). Although these definitions do overlap, telehealth is not limited just to the delivery of services to clients or patients who are unwell but also includes preventative health care practices, education, and administrative activities. The Agency for Healthcare Research and Quality (AHRQ) describes telehealth as the use of information and communication technologies to support patients by delivering health-related services, health information and education, and administrative activities (Dixon, Hook, & McGowan, 2008; Houston & Behl, 2012). Using this definition, telemedicine can be seen as a division or subset of the broader telehealth concept (Constantinescu, 2010; Darkins & Cary, 2000). However, because of the overlap in these definitions, the terms telemedicine and telehealth are sometimes used interchangeably (Baker & Bufka, 2011; Houston & Behl, 2012). Houston and Behl (2012) note that, due to this confusion or lack of consistency, many disciplines in the health field have developed their own terminology to describe the services that are being provided. Some examples include teleradiology, telecardiology, telenursing, and teleaudiology.

The term telepractice was adopted by the American Speech-Language-Hearing Association (ASHA) to be used instead of the terms telemedicine and telehealth. The intended outcome of this was to change the misperception that this model of service delivery relates only to health care or medical settings (ASHA, 2014b). Other terms such as teleaudiology can be used in addition to telepractice. Services delivered by an audiologist are sometimes included in the broader generic term telerehabilitation (American Telemedicine Association, 2010; Smith-Welsh, 1999). Telerehabilitation has been added to the nomenclature to represent the health care disciplines such as speech-language pathology, occupational therapy, and physiotherapy, in addition to audiology, which have all adopted the use of information and communication technologies in the delivery of services (Bauer & Ringel, 1999; Constantinescu, 2010; Maheu et al., 2001).

Although the original aim of these applications was to deliver health-related services at a distance, either by linking the health care provider and the patient or by linking health professionals when they are located in different places (Krumm, 2005; Loane & Wootton, 2001; Rushbrooke, 2012; Swanepoel et al., 2010), it is increasingly observed that this model of service delivery also offers convenient access for clients or patients who may not be at a significant distance from the health care provider. Mobility issues, people who are time poor due to full-time work, and parents with small children are all examples where telehealth services can improve equity of access.

Telepractice in Audiology: Teleaudiology

Teleaudiology can be defined as the utilization of telehealth to deliver audiological diagnostic treatment and management services (Houston & Behl, 2012; *Tele-audiology*, n.d.). Historically, the development of teleaudiology was driven by concerns with access to hearing health care professionals and the struggle that many people with hearing and communication problems face (Crowell, Givens, Jones, Brechtelsbauer, & Yao, 2011). In audiology, there are significant gaps in service provision and, from a global perspective, close to 80% of persons with hearing loss do not have access to hearing health care services because they live in developing countries where audiologists or other hearing health care workers are unavailable (Fagan & Jacobs, 2009; Goulios & Patuzzi, 2008; Swanepoel & Hall, 2010; Swanepoel, Hall, & Biagio, 2011). In addition, the current production of hearing aids meets less than 10% of global need, and fewer than 1 in 40 who need a hearing aid have one. In relation to audiologists, estimates for developing nations are 1:500,000 to 6.25 million and 1:20,000 in developed nations (Abrams, n.d.; Swanepoel et al., 2010; WHO, 2014). Although access for people in rural and remote areas has been a key driver, increasingly it is being acknowledged that access can also be difficult in more urban areas (Nemes, 2010). A shift toward a telepractice model, or a combination of face-to-face and telepractice service provision (i.e., a hybrid model), to populations located in more urban areas is being observed, and this not only has the potential to increase access but may also improve efficiency in the health care system (Swanepoel, 2013).

The term teleaudiology was first used in 1999 by Dr. Gregg Givens in reference to a system being developed at East Carolina University in Greenville, North Carolina. The first audiological test via the Internet was successfully performed in 2000 by Givens, Balch, and Keller (Abrams, n.d.; Nemes, 2010). At the 2009 AudiologyNOW, American Academy of Audiology Annual Convention, Dr. James Hall successfully performed the first transatlantic tele-audiology test from Dallas, Texas, to South Africa (Abrams, n.d.; Nemes, 2010; *Tele-audiology*, n.d.). Since that historic event, the interest in teleaudiology has increased significantly.

Results from the American Speech-Language-Hearing Association, from surveys administered in 2002 and 2014, help to document the growth and increased integration of telepractice in the audiology profession. ASHA surveyed audiologists in 2002 and found that only 12% of audiologists were using some form of telehealth practice at that time (ASHA, 2002; Givens, 2004). In 2014, ASHA's Special Interest Group (SIG) 18 fielded a Web-based survey to both audiologists and speech-language pathologists. Participants were asked if they were currently providing services through telepractice, with 51.9% of respondent audiologists reporting that they were (ASHA, 2014a). Although this growth is very pleasing to observe, this result also highlights the fact that there are a large number of audiologists not utilizing telepractice to deliver services.

The audiology profession is uniquely suited to provide a range of services using telepractice. Today, an audiologist in one location can log in to a remote computer and deliver services at a distance. This is due to the combination of information and communication technology and the technical nature of audiological screening, diagnostic, and rehabilitation equipment. Teleaudiology has the capability of providing services to all age groups across a continuum of care; many audiologists would benefit from considering how a teleaudiology approach could better serve their clients (American Telemedicine Association, 2010; ASHA, 2014a, 2014b; Givens, Blanarovich, Murphy, Simmons, Balch, & Elangovan, 2003; Swanepoel et al., 2011). Many of the teleaudiology applications are explored further in other chapters of this book, as well as discussion about models of service delivery, the need for more research, and methods or models to evaluate and demonstrate the efficacy of telepractice in audiology.

Summary

Reviewing the history of telepractice applications has reinforced the dynamic nature of this type of service delivery. It has also highlighted that real change and innovation are driven by demand and by the health care workers delivering the service, and that, although technology supports this innovation and change, it is simply a tool. Many applications have emerged within telehealth, and teleaudiology is one of these applications. Growth in applications has also resulted in differing terminology to describe the services, and some of the literature suggests that this can be confusing to people accessing the service as well as to policy makers and other stakeholders. Lack of clarity around terminology and corresponding definitions may hinder growth and acceptance. The field of hearing health needs to capitalize on the exponential growth in information and telecommunication networks to ensure greater adoption of telepractice and, ultimately, improved service delivery to those patients who desperately need audiological diagnostic and treatment services.

References

Abrams, H. B. (n.d.). *Are you ready for connected audiology? A survey of attitudes.* PowerPoint presentation for Starkey Hearing Technologies. Retrieved January 3, 2015, from http://www.ncrar.research.va .gov/Education/Conf_2013/Documents/Abrams1.pdf

American Speech-Language-Hearing Association. (2002). *Survey of telepractice use among audiologists and speech-language pathologists.* Retrieved November 20, 2014, from http://www.asha.org/uploaded Files/practice/telepractice/SurveyofTelepractice.pdf

American Speech-Language-Hearing Association. (2014a). *2014 SIG 18 telepractice survey results.* Retrieved December 29, 2014, from http:// www.asha.org/uploadedFiles/ASHA/Practice_Portal/Professional_ Issues/Telepractice/SIG-18-Telepractice-Services-Survey-Results-by-Profession.pdf

American Speech-Language-Hearing Association. (2014b). *Professional issues/telepractice.* Retrieved May 2014 from http://www.asha.org/ Practice-Portal/Professional-Issues/Telepractice/

American Telemedicine Association. (2010). *A blueprint for telemedicine guidelines.* Retrieved March 25, 2014, from http://www.american telemed.org/docs/default-source/standards/a-blueprint-for-telereha bilitation-guidelines.pdf?sfvrsn=4

Armstrong, D. G., Giovinco, N., Joseph, L., Mills, J. L., & Rogers, L. C. (2011). FaceTime for physicians: Using real time mobile phone–based videoconferencing to augment diagnosis and care in telemedicine. *EPlasty, 11,* 212–217.

Baker, D. C., & Bufka, L. F. (2011). Preparing for the telehealth world: Navigating legal, regulatory, reimbursement and ethical issues in an electronic age. *Professional Psychology: Research and Practice, 42(*6), 405–411.

Bashshur, R. L., Reardon, T. G., & Shannon, G. W. (2000). Telemedicine: A new health care delivery system. *Annual Review of Public Health, 21,* 613–637.

Bashshur, R., Shannon, G., Krupinski, E., & Grigsby, J. (2011). The taxonomy of telemedicine. *Telemedicine Journal and e-Health, 17,* 484–494.

Bashshur, R. L., & Shannon, G. W. (2009). *History of telemedicine: Evolution, context and transformation.* New Rochelle, NY: Mary Ann Liebert.

Bauer, J., & Ringel, M. (1999). *Telemedicine and the reinvention of healthcare.* New York, NY: McGraw-Hill.

Benschoter, R. A., Wittson, C. L., & Ingham, C. G. (1965). Teaching and consultation by television: 1. Closed-circuit collaboration. *Journal of Hospital and Community Psychiatry, 16*(3), 99–100.

Brennan, D. (2013). To move telepractice toward the future, we should look to the past. *SIG 18 Perspectives on Telepractice, 3,* 4–8.

Carson, M. K. (2007). *Alexander Graham Bell: Giving voice to the world.* New York, NY: Sterling.

Chakravorty, R. C. (1976). Dr. Alexander Graham Bell: Audiologist and speech therapist. *Archives of Otolaryngology, 102,* 574–575.

Constantinescu, G. (2010). *Disordered speech and voice in Parkinson's disease using a PC-based telerehabilitation system* (Unpublished doctoral thesis). Brisbane, Australia: The University of Queensland.

Craig, D., & Miskelly, F. (2010). *Telehealth and telecare-best practice guide.* Retrieved November 20, 2014, from http://www.bgs.org.uk/ index.php?option=com_content&view=article&id=646:gpgtelecare& catid=12:goodpractice&Itemid=106

Craig, J., & Patterson, V. (2006). Introduction to the practice of telemedicine. In R. Wootton, J. Craig, & V. Patterson (Eds.), *Introduction to telemedicine* (2nd ed., pp. 3–14). London, UK: Royal Society of Medicine Press.

Cohn, E. (2013). SIG 18 "Coordinators column." *SIG 18 Perspectives on Telepractice, 3,* 3.

Crowell, E. S., Givens, D. G., Jones, G. L., Brechtelsbauer, P. B., & Yao, J. (2011). Audiology telepractice in a clinical environment: A communication perspective. *Annals of Otology, Rhinology & Laryngology, 120*(7), 441–447.

Darkins, A. W., & Cary, M. A. (2000). *Telemedicine and telehealth: Principles, policies, performance, and pitfalls.* London, UK: Free Association Books.

Dennis, K. C., Gladden, C. F., & Noe, C. M. (2012). Telepractice in the Department of Veterans Affairs: An overview of the VA telehealth and pilot tele-audiology programs. *Hearing Review.* Retrieved from http://www.hearingreview.com/2012/10/telepractice-in-the-department-of-veterans-affairs/

Dilts, J. D. (1996). *The great road: The building of the Baltimore and Ohio, the nation's first railroad, 1828–1853.* Palo Alto, CA: Stanford University Press.

Dixon, B. E., Hook, J. M., & McGowan, J. J. (2008). *Using telehealth to improve quality and safety: Finding from the AHRQ Portfolio* (Prepared by the AHRQ National Resource Center for Health IT under contract No. 290-04-0016, AHRQ Publication No. 09-00120EF). Rockville, MD: Agency for Healthcare Research and Quality.

Dzenowagis, J. (2009). Bridging the digital divide: Linking health and ICT policy. In R. Wootton, N. G. Patil, E. Richard, R. E. Scott, & K. Ho (Eds.), *Telehealth in the developing world* (pp. 9–26). London, UK: Royal Society of Medicine Press.

Fagan, J. J., & Jacobs, M. (2009). Survey of ENT services in Africa: Need for a comprehensive intervention. *Global Health Action.* doi:10.3402/gha.v2i0.1932. Retrieved December 29, 2014, from http://www.ncbi.nlm.nih.gov/pmc/articles/PMC2779942/

Fatehi, F., & Wootton, R. (2012). Telemedicine, telehealth or e-health? A bibliometric analysis of the trends in the use of these terms. *Journal of Telemedicine and Telecare, 18*(8), 460–464.

Field, M. J. (1996). Evolution and current applications of telemedicine. In M. J. Field (Ed.), *Telemedicine: A guide to assessing telecommunications for health care* (pp. 34–53). Washington, DC: National Academies Press.

Fuchs, M. (1979). Provider attitudes towards STARPAHC: A telemedicine project on the Papago Reservation. *Medical Care, 17*(1), 59–68.

Garshnek, V., & Burkle, F. (1999a). Application of telemedicine and telecommunications to disaster medicine: Historical and future perspectives. *Journal of the American Medical Informatics Society, 6*(1), 26–37.

Garshnek, V., & Burkle, F. (1999b). Telecommunication systems in support of disaster medicine: Applications of basic information pathways. *Annals of Emergency Medicine, 34*, 213–218.

Givens, G. (2004). Telepractice brings new challenges to audiologists. *The ASHA Leader, 9*(10), 21–41.

Givens, G., Blanarovich, A., Murphy, T., Simmons, S., Balch, D., & Elangovan, S. (2003). Internet-based tele-audiometry system for the assessment of hearing: A pilot study. *Telemedicine Journal and e-Health, 9*(4), 375–378.

Givens, G., & Elangovan, S. (2003). Internet application to tele-audiology—"Nothin but Net." *American Journal of Audiology, 12*(2), 59–65.

Goulios, H., & Patuzzi, R. B. (2008). Audiology education and practice from an international perspective. *International Journal of Audiology, 47*, 647–664.

Gunsch, J. (2011). *What is telemedicine?* Conjecture Corporation. Retrieved from http://www.wisegeek.com/what-is-telemedicine.htm

House, A. M., & Roberts, J. M. (1977). Telemedicine in Canada. *Canadian Medical Association Journal, 117*(4), 386–388.

Houston, K. T. (Ed.). (2014). *Telepractice in speech-language pathology.* San Diego, CA: Plural.

Houston, K. T., & Behl, D. (2012). Using telepractice to improve outcomes for children with hearing loss & their families. In *National Centre for hearing assessment and management* (NCHAM@Book). Retrieved November 2014 from http://www.infanthearing.org/ehdi-ebook/2012_ebook/Chapter11.pdf

Houston, K. T., Behl, D., & Walters, K. Z. (2013). Using telepractice to improve outcomes for children with hearing loss & their families. In *National Centre for hearing assessment and management* (NCHAM@Book). Retrieved August 2014 from http://www.infanthearing.org/ehdi-ebook/2013_ebook/18Chapter17UsingTelepractive2013.pdf

Houston, K. T., Fleming, A. M., Brown, K. J., Weinberg, T. R., & Nafe, J. M. (2014). History, definitions and overview of telepractice models. In K. T. Houston (Ed.), *Telepractice in speech-language pathology* (pp. 1–20). San Diego, CA: Plural.

Huurdeman, A. A. (2003). *The worldwide history of telecommunications.* Hoboken, NJ: John Wiley & Sons.

International Telecommunications Union. (2014). *The world in 2014, ICT facts and figures.* Retrieved January 2015 from http://www.itu.int/en/ITU-D/Statistics/Documents/facts/ICTFactsFigures2014-e.pdf

Internet World Stats. (2014). Retrieved May 11, 2014, from http://www.internetworldstats.com/stats.htm

Kamat, V. (2010). *Medical technology telehealth, mobile health, connected health, and now ECare—is there a difference?* Retrieved November 2014 from http://blog.cambridgeconsultants.com/medical-technology/telehealth-mobile-health-connected-health-and-now-ecare-is-there-a-difference/

Kazely, A. S., McLeod, K. A., & Wager, K. A. (2012). Telemedicine in an international context: Definition, use, and future. In N. Menachemi & S. Singh (Eds.), *Health information technology in the international context* (Vol. 12, pp. 143–169). Bingley, UK: Emerald Group.

Krumm, M. (2005). Audiology telepractice moves from theory to treatment. *The ASHA Leader, 45*, 22–23.

Krumm, M. (2007). Audiology telemedicine. *Journal of Telemedicine and Telecare, 13*, 224–229.

Kuo, R. L., Delvecchio, F. C., Babayan, R. K., & Preminger, G. M. (2001). Telemedicine: Recent developments and future applications. *Journal of Endourology, 15*(1), 63–66.

Loane, M., & Wootton, R. (2001). A review of telehealth. Review Telematics Series 3. *Medical Principles Practices, 10*, 163–170.

Maheu, M. M., Whitten, P., & Allen, A. (2001). *E-health, telehealth, and telemedicine: A guide to start-up and success.* San Francisco, CA: Jossey-Bass.

Mun, S. K., & Turner, J. W. (1999). Telemedicine: Emerging e-medicine. *Annual Review of Biomedical Engineering, 1*, 589–610.

Murphy, R. L. H., & Bird, K. T. (1974). Telediagnosis: A new community health resource: Observations on the feasibility of telediagnosis based on 1000 patient transactions. *American Journal of Public Health, 64*(2), 113–119.

Nemes, J. (2010). Tele-audiology, a once-futuristic concept, is growing into a worldwide reality. *The Hearing Journal, 63*(2), 19–24.

Perednia, D. A., & Allen, A. (1995). Telemedicine technology and clinical applications. *Journal of the American Medical Association, 273*(6), 483–488.

Rushbrooke, E. (2012). *Remote MAPping for children with cochlear implants* (Unpublished master's thesis). Brisbane, Australia: The University of Queensland.

Smith-Welsh, T. (1999). *Telemedicine. Telemedicine Network.* Available from http://ocean.st.usm.edu/~w146169/teleweb/telemed.htm

Stanberry, B. (1998a). *The legal and ethical aspects of telemedicine.* London, UK: Royal Society of Medicine Press.

Stredler-Brown, A. (2014). Efficacy of telepractice in speech-language pathology. In K. T. Houston (Ed.), *Telepractice in speech-language pathology* (pp. 21–50). San Diego, CA: Plural.

Swanepoel, D. (2013). 20Q: Audiology to the people—combining technology and connectivity for services by telehealth. *AudiologyOnline*, Article 12183. Retrieved from http://www.audioloyonline.com

Swanepoel, D., Clark, J., Koekemoer, D., Hall, J., Krumm, M., Ferrari, D., . . . Barajas, J.(2010). Telehealth in audiology: The need and potential to reach underserved communities. *International Journal of Audiology, 49*, 195–202.

Swanepoel, D., & Hall, J. (2010). A systematic review of telehealth applications in audiology. *Telemedicine Journal and e-Health, 16*, 181–200.

Swanepoel, D., Hall, J., & Biagio, L. (2011). Tele-audiology offers great promise in reaching underserved people globally. *Hearing*

Views @ Hearing Health Matters. Retrieved April 8, 2014, from http://hearinghealthmatters.org/hearingviews/2011/tele-audiology-offers-great-promise

Tele-audiology. (n.d.). Retrieved September 2014 from http://en.wiki pedia.org/wiki/Tele-audiology

Teleradiology: Historical overview. (n.d). Retrieved November 2014 from http://www.tetradiology.com/newsletter/HistoryofTeleradiology.pdf

van Dyk, L. (2014). A review of telehealth service implementation frameworks. *International Journal of Environment, Research and Public Health, 11,* 1279–1298.

Welsh, T. S. (1999). *Telemedicine.* Telemedicine Network. Retrieved from http://ocean.st.usm.edu/~w146169/teleweb/telemed.htm

Whitten, P., Frances, M., & Collins, B. (1997). Home telenursing in Kansas: Patient's perceptions of users and benefits. *Journal of Telemedicine and Telecare, 3*(Suppl. 1), 67–69.

Wootton, R., Patil, N. G., Scott, R. E., & Ho, K. (2009). Introduction. In R. Wootton, N. G. Patil, R. E. Scott, & K. Ho (Eds.), *Telehealth in the developing world* (p. 285). London, UK: Royal Society of Medicine Press.

World Health Organization. (2014). *Deafness and hearing loss.* Retrieved April 8, 2014, from http://www.who.int/mediacentre/factsheets/fs300/en/

Xiaohui, Y., Han, H., Jiadong, D., Liurong, W., Cheng, L., Xueli, Z., . . . Bleiberg, J. (2013). *mHealth in China and the United States: How mobile technology is transforming healthcare in the world's two largest economies* (Executive summary). Washington, DC: Centre for Technology Innovation at Brookings.

Zundel, K. (1996). Telemedicine: History, applications, and impact on librarianship. *Bulletin of the Medical Library Association, 84*(1), 71–79.

2

Models of Service Delivery: What Should We Consider?

Emma Rushbrooke

Key Points

- Teleaudiology has the potential to improve equity of access to unserved or underserved children and adults seeking audiological services.
- Audiology, as a profession, is uniquely suited to a tele-practice approach.
- There are different models or approaches to telepractice service delivery in audiology.
- Multiple factors may influence implementation of a tele-audiology model of service delivery.
- Planning, validation, and stakeholder engagement are key to successful teleaudiology practice.

Incorporating telepractice into audiological service delivery improves equity of access to hearing health care and may also enable audiologists and other hearing health care professionals to better serve their clients by providing more flexible service options. Current statistics show that there are 360 million people worldwide with disabling hearing loss, including 32 million children (World Health Organization, 2014). There is a shortage of hearing health care professionals in most regions of the world (Swanepoel & Hall, 2010), and this, in conjunction with an increasingly aging population, means that consideration of different models of service delivery, such as teleaudiology, needs to be embraced by professionals in the field.

Audiology is uniquely suited to provide a range of services using telepractice. Today's connectivity technology enables an audiologist in one location to log in to a remote computer and deliver services, at a distance, by linking clinician-to-client or clinician-to-clinician for assessment, intervention, and/or consultation (American Speech-Language-Hearing Association [ASHA], 2014a, 2014b; Swanepoel, Hall, & Biagio, 2011). Although many audiologists may believe that this model of service delivery is not relevant to them, many would benefit from considering how the reality of valid and reliable technological options could be used to better serve their client population and clinical practice by using a teleaudiology framework (Dworsack-Dodge, 2013; Swanepoel et al., 2011). Teleaudiology has the capability of providing "services across the lifespan and across a continuum of care" (American Telemedicine Association, 2010, p. 5), from newborn hearing screening to hearing aid fittings for adults, as well as follow-up support and care for all age groups.

This chapter provides an overview of different approaches to telepractice service delivery and discusses some of the factors that need to be considered to facilitate successful implementation of a telepractice program. Although the focus is on teleaudiology programs, much of the information provided in this chapter can be generalized to other disciplines.

Approaches to Service Delivery Using a Telepractice Model

The models of service delivery are commonly described as either *asynchronous* (store-and-forward) or *synchronous* (real time). These different models relate to the timing of the client-to-clinician or the clinician-to-clinician interactions (Craig & Patterson, 2006; Krumm, Ribera, & Schmiedge, 2005; Krumm & Syms, 2011; Loane & Wootton, 2001; Swanepoel, 2013).

The *asynchronous* model involves images or data being collected and stored at a remote site, and this information is then forwarded or transmitted to a professional/consultant for interpretation and/or review (ASHA, 2014a, 2014b). The asynchronous model is already used in some form by most audiologists such as for electronic medical records, video-otoscopy images transmitted via email or automated audiometry (Biagio, Swanepoel, Adeyemo, Hall, & Vinck, 2013; Biagio, Swanepoel, Laurent, & Lundberg, 2014).

The *synchronous* model allows real-time interaction between the client and clinician, using a variety of technologies such as telephone, email, videoconferencing, webcam, or remote control of a computer-based diagnostic assessment using remote desktop-sharing software. Interactive video is often used with the synchronous model, and this technology enables an essentially face-to-face service using either a computer-based Web camera or a dedicated camera system. There are also different service provision options or paradigms that the clinician may use with interactive video synchronous models. The first involves interactive video to supervise a technician at a remote service site. The technician is trained to perform the test procedures, and the clinician provides diagnostic information and management recommendations to the client once the testing is complete (Krumm & Syms, 2011).

The second incorporates the use of interactive video and remote control software to enable the clinician to test the client from a distance. This approach also has variations that have been described as either *direct connection* or *connection via a facilitator*. Direct connection involves the clinician connecting directly to the client for the delivery of services; this approach is "self-administered" and does not require a support person to be present (Singh, 2013). The connection via a facilitator approach utilizes the same technology as direct connection, with, in addition, a facilitator or support person present to assist with set up of the equipment and provide support throughout the consultation. One example of this approach in audiology is the delivery of remote programming of cochlear implants. Using the connection via a facilitator model, an audiologist is able to program a cochlear implant from a distance in real time, using video and audio communication technology and remote programming software, such as Remote Desktop. This has been reported in a number of publications, and in each case, a trained support person or audiologist was present at the client's site to assist in facilitating the session (Eikelboom et al., 2014; McElveen, Blackburn, Green, McLear, Thimsen, & Wilson, 2010; Psarros, Rushbrooke, & van Wanrooy, 2012; Ramos et al., 2009; Rushbrooke, 2012).

Although some circumstances support the discrete use of either an asynchronous or synchronous approach, clinicians should consider the most effective and efficient model to deliver a specific telepractice service. In many situations, a combination of these models of service delivery will achieve the best outcome (Krumm & Syms, 2011). Both synchronous and asynchronous approaches have been used together successfully in many health-related areas, such as otolaryngology, by using video-otoscopy together with audiogram and tympanometry results (Eikelboom & Atlas, 2004; Eikelboom, Mbao, Coates, Atlas, & Gallop, 2005; Sclafani, Heneghan, Ginsburg, Stern, & Dolitsky, 1997; Syms & Syms, 2001) and also demonstrated in a school-based hearing screening program where remote control software and a Web camera were used to perform pure-tone audiograms. In this example, tympanometry results were viewed via Web camera at the time of screening and then scanned and sent via email for later interpretation by the clinician (Krumm & Syms, 2011; Lancaster, Krumm, Ribera, & Klich, 2008). The combined use of both approaches is called a *hybrid* model, which enables the interaction of both the synchronous and asynchronous models, facilitating a flexible and integrated approach. In audiology, the hybrid model offers the opportunity to deliver a battery of assessments, as highlighted in the school-based program above, and enables the provision of more complete hearing services via telepractice (Krumm & Syms, 2011).

The term *hybrid* is also sometimes used in relation to telerehabilitation, eSupervision, eTraining, and eMentoring, and it refers to a combination of services and/or support delivered by both telepractice and face-to-face modes (Carlin, Carlin, Milam, & Weinberg, 2014). This is an option that has the potential to enhance the follow-up care required after face-to-face consultations in audiological practice.

What Model Should Be Used?

There is no one correct telepractice model of service delivery in audiology, but the implementation of an approach requires careful planning. The decision is dependent on what service is being delivered and the desired outcomes. In addition, connectivity and Internet capability will have an impact on this decision. Consideration of these factors will allow clinicians to decide which model is most suitable and will ultimately enable service delivery that meets the needs of both the client and the clinician. The general expectation is that a telepractice program should deliver services and outcomes that are equivalent to providing the same service in the traditional face-to-face model.

Cuyler and Holland (2012) note that, although telepractice has been utilized for many decades, uptake (that is, adoption) of the approach has not been widespread in the health care industry and that it often has a poor record of implementation. In addition, Zanaboni and Wootton (2012) stated that the uptake of telepractice has been fragmented and has a "patchy history of adoption" and integration into ongoing health care. Although technology is becoming increasingly available to health care professionals, these applications are not yet widely used by audiologists (Krumm et al., 2005; Zanaboni & Wootton, 2012), particularly with regards to computer-based synchronous (real-time) communications. There are many factors noted in the literature that impact the successful implementation of a telepractice model, and they include but are not limited to

- Insufficient planning
- Complicated equipment
- Concerns about cost of equipment
- Confidence with equipment and outcomes
- Poor quality picture and sound quality
- Keeping up to date with technology trends
- The environment or setting
- Inadequate staff training
- Concerns that the outcomes are not the same as for a face-to-face service delivery
- Staff/clinician engagement
- Concerns about privacy
- Professional licensing and reimbursement issues

(Constantinescu, 2010; Craig, Russell, Patterson, & Wootton, 1999; Crutchley, Alvares, & Campbell, 2014; Cuyler & Holland, 2012; Singh, 2013). By further exploring and discussing some of these factors, the author hopes to dispel some of the myths and/or concerns that have been propagated.

Planning

When planning to implement a telepractice program in audiology, the first questions that need to be asked are, "What is the need? Who are the services going to be provided to and how are they going to be delivered?"

Crutchley et al. (2014) recommend some basic steps for setting up a telepractice program. Although these relate to a speech and language pathology telepractice program, they are transferrable and relevant to the audiology discipline. The steps are define, research, plan, promote, implement, evaluate, and adjust. In addition, Cuyler and Holland (2012) suggest that there are three fundamental and interdependent risks that need to be considered in the planning process. These include

1. Technical risks—choosing the right equipment means adequate capability and reliability.
2. Organizational risks—is the organization committed and are the staff engaged?
3. Business risks—the program needs to be cost-effective and sustainable.

The clinician also needs to determine the potential benefits of the program, not only for the client but also for the organization or program. Some programs deliver services to regional and remote locations by sending a visiting specialist out to the client(s). This is not always time- or cost-effective; telepractice may offer an alternative. The Sydney Cochlear Implant Centre in Sydney, Australia, has an established remote cochlear implant program. They provide services to more than 3,000 clients, with 60% of its cochlear implant recipients living outside metropolitan areas. In 2012, the center reported that their program had saved about $200,000 a year in clinic "downtime" by not needing to fly hearing health care specialists to locations where they had established remote log-in facilities (Griffith, 2012). Although this is an extreme case, and in general most audiology services would not fly their clinicians to remote sites, it does demonstrate the potential for cost savings. It has been noted in many papers that there is not enough clear evidence that telepractice is a cost-effective means of delivering services, but Zanaboni and Wootton (2012) note that that there has recently been an increase in the number of economic reviews or evaluations in telepractice or telemedicine. However, they do highlight the fact that information being evaluated is not consistent and that this impacts reliability. Hailey and Jennett (2004) reported that the economic assessment of telepractice service delivery continues to be challenged by the availability of data and analytic resources.

A comprehensive understanding of the resources necessary and a realistic budget are essential requirements in the planning phase of program development (Crutchley et al., 2014; Cuyler & Holland, 2012). If there is a demand for the service, if the technology works well, and if the organizational commitment and engagement are high, then one could surmise that the outcome should be not only good audiological care, but also a positive business result and high user satisfaction. Performing a cost benefit analysis and assessing user satisfaction is an essential component for quality assurance and continuous quality improvement. It is important that more evaluations of the cost-effectiveness of telepractice are performed and that there is clarity about the objective and design of the evaluation (Bergmo, 2009). This will make the study transparent and help readers to decide whether results can apply to their own settings. Also, the development of a framework to better enable consistency in these evaluations would be beneficial. These factors are discussed in more detail in Chapter 3 of this book. In addition, equipment, staff, and the service delivery environment need to be considered in the planning phase, and these are discussed in more detail below.

Equipment

Professional groups and associations in audiology have developed guidelines around teleaudiology and specifications relating to equipment. There is general agreement among these professional bodies that the technology needs to be appropriate for the intervention being provided, as the technology may affect the quality of the teleaudiology service, for example, the audio and video quality. The teleaudiology professional practice standards, developed by Audiology Australia in 2013, cite equipment specifications and practice operations in their guidelines. The guidelines state that Audiology Australia does not separate the standards for teleaudiology from those for a face-to-face audiological service delivery model (Audiology Australia, 2013). This emphasizes the fact that outcomes should not be affected when using a telepractice model and highlights the importance of implementing the appropriate equipment solutions. Audiologists considering a teleaudiology model of service delivery should be knowledgeable about current equipment guidelines promoted by the professional or regulating associations. Listed below are the major professional bodies in Australia, the United States, and Canada:

- Audiology Australia
- American Speech-Language-Hearing Association (ASHA)
- American Academy of Audiology (AAA)
- College of Audiologists and Speech-Language Pathologists of Ontario (CASLPO)

There are many equipment and technology options available, and the right choices will be unique to each program or audiology practice. Some factors that will need to be considered are

- The type of technology to be used
- How the technology will be used (e.g., does it need to be portable?)
- Transmission methods and speed, as all technology systems will be affected by bandwidth
- Network availability and reliability
- Audio and video quality, which must be sufficient to carry out the clinical service application
- Is the equipment user friendly?

Informational Technology Support

Having good informational technology (IT) support in the research, planning, and implementation stage is essential when setting up a model of telepractice service delivery (Crutchley et al.,

2014) and will enable the clinician to address the considerations or concerns listed above. Skilled IT support will assist the clinician in finding reliable and user-friendly equipment solutions, and the IT specialist can also provide recommendations relating to the infrastructure. For example, teleconferencing software requires sufficient bandwidth to enable quality real time face-to-face sessions. Consultation with an IT specialist will ensure that the infrastructure capabilities meet the minimum requirements necessary for a quality service delivery. A lack of technological compatibility may be a barrier to connecting to sites with different hardware, software, and bandwidth speeds (ASHA, 2014a, 2014b). Audiologists will need to consider the possibility that a financial outlay may be required to upgrade the infrastructure. Establishing a relationship with an IT specialist to oversee the planning and implementation of a teleaudiology service will enhance outcomes and efficiency and increase confidence in the technology solutions.

Taking Advantage of Technological Trends

Advances in technology, especially in the past decade, have greatly influenced the health care industry and provide a bridge between clients and clinicians (Ribera, 2005; Swanepoel & Hall, 2010). The purchase cost of equipment may be a concern for many clinicians or programs, but the rapid changes and advances in technology have not only enabled more options but have also resulted in a reduction in the price of the technology. This means that the capital costs to set up a teleaudiology program are becoming much more affordable and, therefore, the cost of equipment should be less of a barrier (Denton & Gladstone, 2005).

As previously noted, the use of computer-based synchronous (real-time) communications are not yet widely or regularly used in audiological service delivery. However, the literature does note that an area that has seen growth, in the more general health care industry, is in the use of videoconferencing technology, which suggests greater acceptance of this as a valid approach to service delivery. Videoconferencing can enable access to high-quality health care services, and the cost of many of these systems is reducing, thus making them more accessible

(Armstrong, Giovinco, Joseph, Mills, & Rogers, 2011; Xiaohui et al., 2013). Videoconferencing can be delivered through a dedicated fixed system or via a personal computer using teleconferencing software.

The disadvantages of a dedicated videoconferencing system are less flexibility and mobility, services can be delivered only between fixed sites, and this may not meet the needs or goals of all teleaudiology services. The mobility of a computer-based teleconferencing option allows greater flexibility, as services can be delivered from multiple sites, which should lead to increased accessibility and, in some cases, services can even be offered in the client's home or work environment. These technology options offer additional solutions for clinical practice and may contribute to time and cost saving for those clients who live a distance away from their service clinic. If services, such as providing support and rehabilitation after hearing aid or cochlear implant fitting, can be delivered using telepractice, this reduces the burden of travel and associated costs and, for some clients, time away from work and family commitments.

Other technology options such as FaceTime and Skype offer a simple and accessible solution for hearing health care providers to communicate across large geographic areas at a much lower cost (Armstrong et al., 2011; Xiaohui et al., 2013). A platform such as Skype is easily accessible, easy to use, and familiar, as it is commonly used by the general public. It also provides a videoconferencing option at no cost. However, although this technology has some advantages, privacy and security may be a concern due to the level of encryption used by a platform such as Skype. Encryption is the process of encoding information or data in such a way that only those who are authorized will be able to access it. The level of encryption used by different technology options needs to be considered by the clinician, as it may impact the technology options that can be considered. Regulations will vary, depending on which country and/or organization you are practicing in, with regard to the privacy protection requirements. The clinician should research this area and develop a firm understanding of these requirements, regulations, and preferred practices when planning a program or service. There are a number of options for obtaining a secure Internet connection during telepractice. These include the use of encryption, passwords, connection via a virtual private network (VPN), and hardware/ software firewalls (ASHA, 2014b).

Technology is moving and changing at a very fast pace, and therefore teleaudiology programs will need to evolve in order to take advantage of these trends (Anne, Kelly, & Houston, 2013). In today's world, increased access to the Internet and the tremendous growth in the use of Web-based technology are providing global opportunities for telepractice implementation that did not previously exist. Cloud computing has applications for both synchronous and asynchronous telepractice and allows clinicians "to share information easily and from multiple devices" (Anne et al., 2013). Also, most mobile devices, such as tablet computers and smartphones, interact with the cloud, and this creates new opportunities (Anne et al., 2013). Mobile devices are now becoming more prevalent due to greater access to cellular networks; telepractice services delivered via these types of technology are known as mHealth (i.e., mobile health). Swanepoel and Hall (2010) note that this mode of delivery is very exciting, as it uses consumer-grade hardware, which means greater access and wider mobility. According to the World Bank, 90% of the world's population has access to a mobile phone signal, and three quarters of the world has mobile phone access. As well, the developing world is now more mobile than the developed world (Edwards, 2012). These factors, combined with global trends, will influence and benefit service delivery now and into the future. In order for audiologists to take advantage of these trends, they must be cognizant of these advances and remain current with research in the field. Future directions of teleaudiology are discussed in Chapter 11.

Professional Licensing and Reimbursement for Telepractice Services

Professional licensing processes for audiologists vary from country to country, and telepractice, as a service delivery model, may be recognized and supported through clearly written guidelines and policies. Conversely, in other countries or professional licensing bodies, telepractice may be viewed with skepticism, and professionals attempting to provide these services may face additional challenges. That is, the audiologist's or hearing health care provider's professional license may influence and limit the scope of services that can be delivered through telepractice. For example, licensure remains a challenge for telepractice providers in the United States. According to ASHA, only 18 states and the District of Columbia have addressed telepractice in their laws, regulations, or policy statements, but this situation is slowly changing. Considerable variability exists among states in terminology and the specificity of existing regulations. Providing telepractice services across state lines requires securing and maintaining licensure in both states. This requirement is often cost prohibitive and requires considerable administrative support and oversight. For these reasons, providers usually limit their services to their home state. Currently, several organizations (e.g., the Federation of State Medical Boards, American Telemedicine Association) are exploring and advocating systems of licensure portability that remove barriers and improve access to interstate telepractice services.

Reimbursement for services continues to be a challenge for providers who are utilizing telepractice models, especially in those countries that require third-party or insurance coverage/payment for services. Brown, Brannon, and Romanow (2010) describe some of these challenges in the United States and the fact that as telepractice in health care continues to grow, Medicare and Medicaid either do not allow telepractice or restrict reimbursement for audiological and speech-language services provided through a telepractice model. Although this is disheartening, some states have modified their state regulations regarding Medicaid or have passed legislation that defines how reimbursement can occur. Although not perfect, practitioners should investigate if and how these services have been addressed. Changes in health care funding paradigms beyond the traditional fee-for-service model should also allow coverage for audiology and speech-language services. In those countries where universal health care is a standard, reimbursement issues may not be a problem. However, equipment, training, and other costs may impact the professional's ability to provide appropriate telepractice services.

Promoting Natural Interactions

Although technology offers great opportunities for service delivery, it is important for hearing health care professionals to be aware of the potential impact that technology may have on the client appointment or consultation and the ability to develop a good rapport with the client. Siden (1998) used a focus group method and qualitative approach to assess community and provider needs in a telepractice project. Both positive and negative attitudes were reported from this group, but the themes that were highlighted by all the participants were "uncertainty" and "trust." Uncertainty related to some aspects of the technology, and trust related to both the technology and the professional or health care worker providing the service. These responses highlight the need to have confidence in the technology. The audiologist needs to be confident in utilizing the equipment and providing a meaningful explanation of the technology to the client prior to the appointment. By so doing, the audiologist is more likely to increase client trust, and this in turn may improve efficiency (Rushbrooke, 2012; Siden, 1998).

With regard to the ability to have natural interactions, teleaudiology can be informed by studies in the area of psychiatry and social work (Bashshur, Mandil, & Shannon, 2002; Bear, Jacobson, Aaronson, & Hanson, 1997; De Las Cuevas, Arredondo, Cabrera, Sulzenbacher, & Meise, 2006; Elford et al., 2000; Elford, White, St. John, Maddigan, & Ghandi, 2001; McCarty & Clancy, 2002; Melaka & Edirippulige, 2009; Ruskin et al., 2004). Videoconferencing (VC) technology is integral to the delivery of telepsychiatry services, because it enables real-time, interactive, two-way audio and video communication in full color (De Las Cuevas et al., 2006; Melaka & Edirippulige, 2009). Bashshur et al. (2002) reported that telepsychiatry is one of the most commonly used applications involving real-time consultations with a high degree of "concordance in diagnostic reliability between telepsychiatric and in-person consults" (p. 96). Ruskin et al. (2004) conducted a large-scale randomized controlled trial and found no significant differences between telepsychiatry and face-to-face consultations.

In addition, Elford et al. (2000) measured satisfaction with a telepsychiatry program in a participant group consisting of 18 children and 23 parents. They reported that, overall, children involved in the study were positive about the VC system that was used, and an equal proportion favored VC and face-to-face assessment. The majority of parents reported that their preference would be to use telepsychiatric services as an alternative to traveling to access care. They also noted that they were generally happy with their ability to speak with and listen to the psychiatrist in the session clearly. These findings are significant in relation to teleaudiology; a psychiatrist needs to observe emotional and behavioral responses similar to what would be required for audiological behavioral assessment. The ability to development a good rapport with the client for provision of test results, counseling, and recommendations is also essential and supported by these findings (Rushbrooke, 2012). Bashshur et al. (2002) also noted that high-quality images (requiring higher bandwidth) are essential for these positive outcomes.

It has also been suggested that client confidence in a telepractice service may improve if clinicians delivering the service are able to display an empathetic and warm manner and maintain good eye contact throughout the session (Constantinescu, 2010; Hill et al., 2006; Hughes, 2001; Miller, 2001; Rushbrooke, 2012; Waite, Cahill, Theodoros, Busuttin, & Russell, 2006). Telepractice systems that are user-friendly and allow the participants to interact in ways that are similar to face-to-face sessions (ASHA, 2005; Denton & Gladstone, 2005) should improve user satisfaction and achieve more positive outcomes.

Environment

Telepractice can be delivered in a variety of settings, which could include schools, hospitals, community health centers, medical and outpatient clinics, universities, homes of clients, senior citizen care facilities, childcare centers, and workplace settings. There are no inherent limits to where telepractice can be implemented, as long as the services comply with national, state, institutional, and professional regulations and policies (ASHA, 2014a,

2014b). Audiologists will be guided to some extent by the type of service or test being administered. Attention to the service delivery environment is an essential component of a successful teleaudiology service, as it is important to ensure confidentiality, comfort, safety, and privacy during the teleaudiology session (ASHA, 2014a). Where appropriate, both the local and remote testing environments should be audited for occupational health and safety (Audiology Australia, 2013).

Considerations as to whether a dedicated space is required will again depend on the type of service being delivered. Having a dedicated space will ensure that the equipment setup and environment will be maintained at a certain standard and available whenever required. However, the disadvantage of a dedicated space is that it restricts the function of the room and may impact room utilization, and this may not be a viable option for all services or locations.

Some of the current applications for teleaudiology include

- Remote cochlear implant programming
- Hearing aid fittings and verification
- Infant hearing screening
- Diagnostic hearing assessments
- Teleotoscopy
- Speech-in-noise testing
- Internet-based treatment for tinnitus
- Counseling
- Habilitation and rehabilitation

Room lighting and layout combined with positioning of the client should help to facilitate the optimal use of the video and audio transmission. Furniture should be comfortable and appropriate for the age and needs of the client and for the service being delivered. Room acoustics will also need to meet certain requirements depending on the service being delivered. Internet connectivity is obviously essential to good outcomes, and this should be checked prior to the commencement of a session. This last point highlights the importance of preplanning and ensuring that all equipment and materials required for the session are available and working prior to the commencement of the session.

Participants in the session should always be aware of who is in the room at both the remote and testing audiologist sites. Permission should always be obtained for an additional clinician or visitor in one of the locations. If a session is going to be recorded, permission for this must also be obtained.

Stakeholder Engagement

People variables have a major impact on the successful implementation of a telepractice program, and the introduction of a teleaudiology program will require organizational change. It is essential that all stakeholders (staff, client, and workplace/ organization) are engaged and supportive. Planning and a clear vision will assist. However, any concerns need to be followed up and alleviated quickly. We have already discussed the importance of choosing the right equipment and the need for it to be user-friendly. Singh (2013) reported that many clinicians might assume that the attitudes of the client toward teleaudiology are what matters most. Singh (2013) noted, however, that the literature does not suggest this but rather that acceptance by clinicians is a key factor. Whitten and Mackert (2005) confirmed this, describing the practitioner or provider as "the most important initial gatekeeper for success with telemedicine interventions" (p. 518).

One of the other influencing factors noted earlier in this chapter was the question as to whether the outcomes are the same when a service is delivered via telepractice. Although there are limited empirical studies on teleaudiology, a systematic review by Swanepoel and Hall (2010) demonstrated reliable and effective applications of teleaudiology with comparable outcomes to face-to-face delivery. As shown previously, the field of audiology can also be informed by research looking at telepractice delivery in other health and allied health disciplines.

It is the author's experience that, in the implementation phase of a telepractice program, a pilot study that compares results obtained remotely versus face-to-face delivery within the clinic is very useful. This can often be done initially room-to-room in the clinic as a "proof-of-concept" evaluation. Commencing with a pilot program allows the clinician to troubleshoot any issues, assess reliability, and perform some initial validation of outcomes. By doing this, participant confidence will be increased when the program is implemented more fully and across greater distances and under "real-world" conditions.

One of the key factors to successful outcomes is the support person or facilitator at the remote site. This is the person who manages the technology at the client point of contact and who may also assist in the service delivery. For example, the support person may assist with distraction when remotely programming a child's cochlear implant (Eikelboom et al., 2014; Psarros et al., 2012; Rushbrooke, 2012). The development of procedure guidelines, education, and training are essential for the ongoing sustainability and success of a teleaudiology program. The support person should possess the following qualities: flexibility, ability to establish a rapport with the client, willingness to learn, some technical skills, and the ability to stay calm and assist with troubleshooting, if technical or connectivity issues occur.

The development of procedure guidelines is also essential for all the audiological staff who will be involved in the teleaudiology program as well as training and education. Some of the qualities that you may consider when selecting staff include

- Has reasonable knowledge of computers and other equipment being used
- Can troubleshoot video and audio equipment and remain calm
- Can attend to technology while conducting the session
- Has organizational skills and the ability to assist with preplanning

Consistent policies and procedures and appropriate training should increase confidence for participants involved in telepractice service delivery.

It is also important to highlight the benefit of evaluation of the satisfaction of all participants (i.e., clients and professionals). This type of evaluation will enable continuous quality improvement of individual teleaudiology programs. Swanepoel and Hall (2010) noted that there is very limited information available related to client and clinician perceptions of teleaudiology services. The level of professional and patient satisfaction with telehealth services is likely to impact the willingness to adopt this approach into clinical practice (Constantinescu, 2010; Craig et al., 1999). Careful planning, communication, and staged implementation should foster stakeholder confidence and satisfaction in the teleaudiology service.

Summary

Teleaudiology can be used across a wide range of audiological services, utilizing different models of delivery. It has the potential to improve access to unserved and underserved populations, and the fast rate of technological change and expanding global connectivity offer tremendous opportunities in the field. Research and validation of telepractice models need to be encouraged, and audiologists should ensure that the standards of service delivery are maintained and equivalent to those delivered face-to-face. The cost benefits also need further evaluation. Analysis of the cost benefit together with outcomes data and validation research will encourage a wider adoption of teleaudiology services. As the technological landscape continues to change and evolve, more audiologists need to investigate and embrace this approach to service delivery.

References

American Speech-Language-Hearing Association. (2005). *Knowledge and skills needed by audiologists providing clinical services via telepractice.* Retrieved September 25, 2008, from http://www.asha.org/telepractice.htm

American Speech-Language-Hearing Association. (2014a). *Information about telepractice in audiology.* Retrieved March 25, 2014, from http://www.asha.org/practice/telepractice/

American Speech-Language-Hearing Association. (2014b). *Telepractice overview.* Retrieved April 4, 2014, from http://www.asha.org/Practice-Portal/Professional-Issues/Telepractice/

American Telemedicine Association. (2010). *A blueprint for telemedicine guidelines*. Retrieved March 25, 2014, from http://www.american telemed.org/docs/default-source/standards/a-blueprint-for-telereha bilitation-guidelines.pdf?sfvrsn=4

Anne, M. F., Kelly, J. B., & Houston, T. (2013) Putting the "tele-" in telepractice. *SIG 18, Perspectives on Telepractice, 3*, 9–15. Retrieved March 15, 2014, from http://sig18perspectives.pubs.asha.org/article .aspx?articleid=1811796

Armstrong, D. G., Giovinco, N., Mills, J. L., & Rogers, L. C. (2011). Face-Time for physicians: Using real time mobile phone–based videoconferencing to augment diagnosis and care in telemedicine. *EPlasty, 11*, 212–217.

Audiology Australia. (2013). *Professional Practice Standards Part B: Clinical standards, Version 1: July 2013*. Retrieved 2014 from http:// www.audiology.asn.au/

Bashshur, R. L., Mandil, S. H., & Shannon, G. W. (2002). Executive summary. *Telemedicine Journal and e-Health, 8*(1), 95–107.

Bear, D., Jacobson, G., Aaronson, S., & Hanson, A. (1997). Telemedicine in psychiatry: Making the dream reality (Letter to the editor). *American Journal of Psychiatry, 154*, 884–885.

Bergmo, T. (2009). Can economic evaluation in telemedicine be trusted? A systematic review of the literature. *Cost Effectiveness and Resource Allocation, 7*, 18.

Biagio, L., Swanepoel, D., Adeyemo, A., Hall, J. W. III, & Vinck, B. (2013). Asynchronous video-otoscopy by a telehealth facilitator. *Telemedicine and e-Health, 19*, 252–258.

Biagio, L., Swanepoel, D., Laurent, C., & Lundberg, T. (2014). Video-otoscopy recordings for diagnosis of childhood ear disease using telehealth at primary health care level. *Journal of Telemedicine and Telecare, 20*(6), 300–306.

Brown, J., Brannon, J., & Romanow, K. (2010). Reimbursement for Tele-speech. *SIG 3 Perspectives on Voice and Voice Disorders, 20*, 16–21.

Carlin, H., Carlin, E., Milam, J., & Weinberg, T. (2014). eSupervision and eMentoring: Professional development for current and future professionals. In K. T. Houston (Ed.), *Telepractice in speech-language pathology* (pp. 209–235). San Diego, CA: Plural.

Constantinescu, G. (2010). *Disordered speech and voice in Parkinson's disease using a PC-based telerehabilitation system* (Unpublished doctoral thesis). Brisbane, Australia: The University of Queensland.

Craig, J., & Patterson, V. (2006). Introduction to the practice of telemedicine. In R. Wootton, J. Craig, & V. Patterson (Eds.), *Introduction to telemedicine* (2nd ed., pp. 3–14). London, UK: Royal Society of Medicine Press.

Craig, J., Russell, C., Patterson, V., & Wootton, R. (1999). User satisfaction with realtime teleneurology. *Journal of Telemedicine and Telecare, 5,* 237–241.

Crutchley, S., Alvares, R., & Campbell, M. (2014). Getting started: Building a successful telepractice program. In K. T. Houston (Ed.), *Telepractice in speech-language pathology* (pp. 51–81). San Diego, CA: Plural.

Cuyler, R., & Holland, D. (2012). *Implementing telemedicine.* Bloomington, IN: Xlibris.

De Las Cuevas, C., Arredondo, M. T., Cabrera, M. F., Sulzenbacher, H., & Meise, U. (2006) Randomized clinical trial of telepsychiatry through videoconference versus face-to-face conventional psychiatric treatment. *Telemedicine and e-Health, 12*(3), 341–350.

Denton, D. R., & Gladstone, V. S. (2005). Ethical and legal issues related to telepractice. *Seminars in Hearing, 26*(1), 43–52.

Dworsack-Dodge, M. (2013). Teleaudiology for enhanced hearing care: Merging traditional face-to-face with face time. *Beyhearing News.* Retrieved April 8, 2014, from http://beyhearing.com/news/d22

Edwards, L. (2012). *Three quarters of the globe have mobile phone access.* Nokia SA Blog. Retrieved April 10, 2014, from http://blog.nokia.co.za/opinions/three-quarters-of-the-globe-have-mobile-phone-access/

Eikelboom, R., & Atlas, M. (2004). Tele-otology for children with chronic ear disease. In R. Wootton & J. Batch (Eds.), *Telepediatrics: Telemedicine and child health* (pp. 153–173). Oxford, UK: Royal Society of Medicine.

Eikelboom, R., Jayakody, D., Swanepoel, D., Chang, S., & Atlas, M. (2014). Validation of remote mapping of cochlear implants. *Journal of Telemedicine and Telecare.* Advance online publication.

Eikelboom, R. H., Mbao, M. N., Coates, H. L., Atlas, M. D., & Gallop, M. A. (2005). Validation of tele-otology to diagnose ear disease in children. *International Journal of Pediatric Otorhinolaryngology, 69,* 739–744.

Elford, D. R., White, H., St. John, K., Maddigan, B., & Ghandi, M. (2001). A prospective satisfaction study and cost analysis of a pilot child telepsychiatry service in Newfoundland. *Journal of Telemedicine and Telecare, 7,* 73–81.

Elford, R., White, H., Bowering, R., Ghandi, A., Maddigan, B., & St. John, K. (2000). A randomized, controlled trial of child psychiatric assessments conducted using videoconferencing. *Journal of Telemedicine and Telecare, 6,* 73–82.

Griffith, C. (2012, November 27). Remote servicing helps spread word to the deaf: Technology is bringing cochlear implants to the developing world. *The Australian.*

Hailey, D., & Jennett, P. (2004). The need for economic evaluation of telemedicine to evolve: The experience in Alberta, Canada. *Telemedicine Journal of E-Health*, *10*(1), 71–76.

Hill, A., Theodoros, D. G., Russell, T. G., Cahill, L. M., Ward, E. C., & Clark, K. M. (2006). An Internet-based telerehabilitation system for the assessment of motor speech disorders: A pilot study. *American Journal of Speech-Language Pathology*, *15*(1), 45–56.

Hughes, E. M. (2001). Communication skills for telehealth interactions. *Home Healthcare Nurse*, *19*(8), 469–472.

Krumm, M., Ribera, J., & Schmiedge, J. (2005). Using a telehealth medium for objective hearing testing: Implications for supporting rural universal newborn hearing screening programs. *Seminars in Hearing*, *26*, 3–12.

Krumm, M., & Syms, M. (2011). Teleaudiology. *Otolaryngologic Clinics of North America*, *44*(6), 1297–1304.

Lancaster, P., Krumm, M., Ribera, J., & Klich, R. (2008). remote hearing screenings via telehealth in a rural elementary school. *American Journal of Audiology*, *17*, 114–122.

Loane, M., & Wootton, R. (2001). A review of telehealth. Review Telematics Series 3. *Medical Principles and Practice*, *10*, 163–170.

McCarty, D., & Clancy, C. (2002). Telehealth: Implications for social work practice. *Social Work*, *47*(2), 153–163.

McElveen, J. T., Blackburn, E. L., Green, D., McLear, P. W., Thimsen, D. J., & Wilson, B. S. (2010). Remote programming of cochlear implants: A telecommunication model. *Otology and Neurotology*, *31*(7), 1035–1040.

Melaka, A., & Edirippulige, S. (2009) *Psych-technology: A systematic review of the telepsychiatry literature*. Centre for Online Health, The University of Queensland. Retrieved November 2014 from http://www.priory.com/printer_friendly.php

Miller, E. (2001). Telemedicine and doctor-patient communication: An analytical survey of the literature. *Journal of Telemedicine and Telecare*, *7*, 1–17.

Psarros, C., Rushbrooke, E., & van Wanrooy, E. (2012, July). *Telemedicine in audiology: Cochlear implant mapping*. Workshop presented at the Audiology Australia 20th National Conference, Adelaide, South Australia.

Ramos, A., Rodriguez, C., Martinez-Beneyto, P., Perez, D., Gault, A., Falcon, J.-C., & Boyle, P. (2009). Use of telemedicine in the remote programming of cochlear implants. *Acta Oto-Laryngologica*, *129*, 533–540.

Ribera, J. (2005). Interjudge reliability and validation of telehealth applications of the hearing in noise test. *Seminars in Hearing*, *26*, 13–18.

Rushbrooke, E. (2012). *Remote mapping for children with cochlear implants* (Unpublished master's thesis). Brisbane, Australia: The University of Queensland.

Ruskin, P. E., Silver-Aylaian, M., Kling, M. A., Reed, S. A., Bradham, D. D., & Hebel, J. R. (2004). Treatment outcomes in depression: Comparison of remote treatment through telepsychiatry to in-person treatment. *American Journal of Psychiatry, 161,* 1471–1476.

Sclafani, A. P., Heneghan, C., Ginsburg, J., Stern, J. C., & Dolitsky, J. N. (1997). Teleconsultation in otolaryngology: Live versus "store-and-forward" consultations. *Otolaryngology-Head and Neck Surgery, 120,* 62–72.

Siden, H. B. (1998). A qualitative approach to community and provider needs assessment in a telehealth project. *Telemedicine Journal, 4,* 225–235.

Singh, G. (2013). *Teleaudiology: Are patients and practitioners ready for it?* Retrieved April 18, 2014, from http://www.phonakpro.com/content/dam/phonak/gc_hq/b2b/en/events/2013/chicago/Singh_SF_2013_Teleaudiology.pdf

Swanepoel, D. (2013). 20Q: Audiology to the people—combining technology and connectivity for services by telehealth. *Audiology Online,* Article 12183. Retrieved from http://www.audioloyonline.com

Swanepoel, D., & Hall, J. (2010). A systematic review of telehealth applications in audiology. *Telemedicine Journal and e-Health, 16,* 181–200.

Swanepoel, D., Hall, J., & Biagio, L. (2011). Tele-audiology offers great promise in reaching underserved people globally. *Hearing Views @ Hearing Health Matters.* Retrieved April 8, 2014, from http://hearinghealthmatters.org/hearingviews/2011/tele-audiology-offers-great-promise

Syms, M., & Syms, C. (2001). The regular practice of telemedicine in otolaryngology. *Archives of Otolaryngology-Head and Neck Surgery, 127,* 333–336.

Waite, M., Cahill, L. M., Theodoros, D. G., Busuttin, S., & Russell, T. G. (2006). A pilot study of online assessment of childhood speech disorders. *Journal of Telemedicine and Telecare, 12*(Suppl. 3), 92–94.

Whitten, P., & Mackert, M. (2005). Addressing telehealth's foremost barrier: Provider as initial gatekeeper. *International Journal of Technology Assessment in Health Care, 21*(4), 517–521.

World Health Organization. (2014). *Deafness and hearing loss.* Retrieved April 8, 2014, from http://www.who.int/mediacentre/factsheets/fs300/en/

Xiaohui, Y., Han, H., Jiadong, D., Liurong, W., Cheng, L., Xueli, Z., . . . Bleiberg, J. (2013). *mHealth in China and the United States: How mobile technology is transforming healthcare in the world's two largest economies* (Executive summary). Washington, DC: Centre for Technology Innovation at Brookings.

Zanaboni, P., & Wootton, R. (2012). Adoption of telemedicine: From pilot stage to routine delivery. *BMC Medical Informatics and Decision Making, 12*, 1.

3

Evaluating the Benefits of a Telepractice Model

Colleen Psarros and Catherine M. McMahon

Key Points

- Ongoing evidence-based research in telepractice is necessary given its dynamic nature.
- Qualitative and quantitative evaluation of telepractice in audiology is a multifaceted process, including a range of stakeholders.
- Ongoing evaluation of telepractice is required to facilitate the implementation into models of service delivery (MOSD) by removing existing barriers.

"To best promote and expand the future of telepractice, we should continue to innovate technology, advocate for changes in reimbursement and licensing, collect strong research data, and collaborate to share our successes and our failures" (Brennan, 2013, p. 4).

Access to health care and rehabilitation programs is problematic for individuals living in rural and remote areas, and significant inequalities in health are evident (Williams, May, Mair, Mort, & Gask, 2003). Improved access for these populations, combined with the aging population, will place a significant economic burden on the health care system. Thus, it is likely that eHealth, mHealth (mobile health), and telepractice will become more common models of health care, health service delivery, and rehabilitation, driven by consumer need and organizational outreach. Evaluating new models of health care and their delivery systems is important and multifactorial.

The multifactorial model for evaluation of telepractice developed by the authors underpins this chapter (Figure 3–1). Telepractice evaluation requires consideration of effectiveness of clinical outcomes, and the quality of outcomes, while remaining in compliance with relevant privacy acts and legislation, and efficiencies as detailed in cost-effectiveness, satisfaction of stakeholders, timeliness of service, access, and ease of implementation (Ruckdaschel, Reiher, Rohrbacher, & Nagel, 2006). Effectiveness and efficiencies must at least emulate those found in traditional models of service delivery (MOSD) involving key stakeholders on site within the clinic. The overarching assumption when using telepractice is that the service provided will be as efficient and as effective as a face-to-face service and will adhere to a code of ethics and scope of practice (Cohn & Carson, 2012).

Telepractice is defined by the World Health Organization (WHO, 2010, p. 9) as "the delivery of health care services, where distance is a critical factor, by all health care professionals using information and communication technologies for the exchange of valid information for diagnosis, treatment and prevention of disease and injuries, research and evaluation, and for the continuing education of health care providers, all in the interests of advancing the health of individuals and their communities." A telepractice model encompasses both eHealth and mHealth. The WHO (2011) defines eHealth as the transfer of health care and health resources through electronic means (p. 1). There is no standardized definition of mHealth, but the Global Observatory for eHealth considers mHealth as health supported by mobile devices, including mobile phones, patient monitoring devices, personal digital assistants, or wireless devices (WHO, 2011). More specifically for the purposes of this chapter, mHealth includes mobile telemedicine, which uses a mobile device through voice, text, imaging, videos, and data to communicate or provide consultations, particularly used in the management of chronic diseases. To reinforce this assumption, clinical practice standards should not separate telepractice from other practice standards. For example, the Audiology Australia standards for documentation, safety, equipment, and settings for telepractice are consistent with all MOSD in audiology (Audiology Australia, 2013).

The telepractice model assumes access, support and implementation of technology is in place. Telepractice as a method of service delivery requires consideration and evaluation as follows:

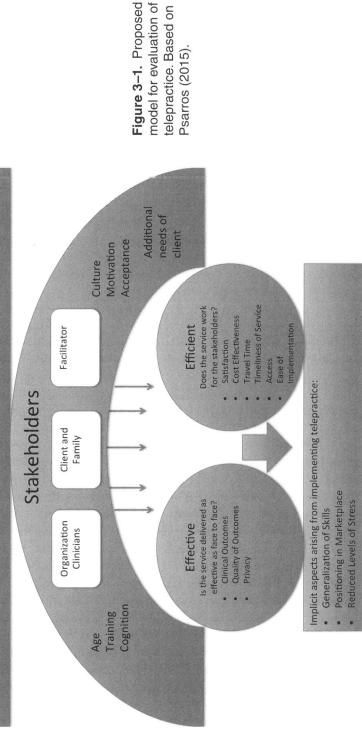

Figure 3–1. Proposed model for evaluation of telepractice. Based on Psarros (2015).

Stakeholders

Organization Clinicians

Client and Family

Facilitator

Age
Training
Cognition

Culture
Motivation
Acceptance

Additional needs of client

Effective

Is the service delivered as effective as face to face?
- Clinical Outcomes
- Quality of Outcomes
- Privacy

Efficient

Does the service work for the stakeholders?
- Satisfaction
- Cost Effectiveness
- Travel Time
- Timeliness of Service
- Access
- Ease of Implementation

Implicit aspects arising from implementing telepractice:
- Generalization of Skills
- Positioning in Marketplace
- Reduced Levels of Stress

The immediate and longer term benefits to all stakeholders involved, including the individual, (i.e., the patient), his or her family, the community, and the organizations involved, will be influenced by the effectiveness and efficiencies of a telepractice model of audiological service delivery. Evaluation of each of these aspects is needed to provide an evidence base for the effectiveness of this approach so that informed decisions can be made by organizations and policy makers about its need, viability, and longer term sustainability. This review focuses on those elements needed for evaluating telepractice that, in turn, can be applied to eHealth and mHealth, which have been less well discussed in the literature.

Current Status of Telepractice in Audiology

There is common agreement in the literature that telepractice can be applied to deliver remote clinical practice, facilitate training and mentoring using best-practice educational models, and enhance interprofessional health care and research collaboration (Swanepoel & Hall, 2010). Telepractice has a clear role in providing services in rural and other underserved areas by reducing travel time and cost, as well as minimizing disruptions to work and educational commitments (Eikelboom, Jayakody, Swanepoel, Chang, & Atlas, 2014; Stith, Stredler-Brown, Greenway, & Kahn, 2012). Additionally, professional up-skilling, training, mentoring, and supervision can be delivered using the same technology, which facilitates adherence to standard models of clinical practice for the professional (Hughes et al., 2012). This reduces the risk of relying on the generalizability of skills learned in a classroom to the professional's clinical practice (see Chapter 9, this volume, for further discussion of telepractice and professional development). Rushbrooke (Chapter 2, this volume) discusses the potential for telepractice to be incorporated into a range of audiological service delivery models. Cameron, Bashshur, Halbritter, Johnson, and Cameron (1998) observed that the "vast majority of telemedicine systems in the US have yet to achieve their full potential in serving their target population and are operating well below capacity" (p. 125).

The landscape has changed significantly with the adoption of telepractice in the areas of psychiatry (Norman, 2006), chronic management of clients in cardiology (Klersy et al., 2011), and speech-language pathology (Stedler-Brown, 2014; Lewis, Packman, Onslow, Simpson, & Jones, 2008; Theodoros et al., 2006), and more closely aligned to hearing health care in the habilitation of children with hearing and vision loss (Blaiser, Edwards, Behl, & Munoz, 2012; Duncan, 2008). Yet, there has certainly been little uptake in the adoption of telepractice in hearing health care worldwide, which may be due, at least in part, to the lack of evidence and other barriers such as financial implications, organizational approaches, and the absence of clear implementation guidelines. A survey by the WHO on the uptake of telemedicine with their member states showed that cost, infrastructure, and lack of information were the main barriers. Proof of the benefits of telepractice methods is required to increase stakeholder confidence in this approach and to provide a clear evidence base to enable wider integration of a telepractice model in audiology.

Defining the Questions for Evaluating Telepractice—The Importance of Evidence-Based Practice

Identification of the need for telepractice as a model of service delivery requires careful consideration of whether it is advantageous over others available and more easily achievable MOSD. Overall, establishment of a solid evidence base is needed to ensure the appropriate service delivery model is chosen.

Evidence-based research requires a triadic interaction between research evidence, the clinician's experience and expertise, and client preferences and goals (Wong & Hickson, 2012). In telepractice, an additional stakeholder group, the facilitator, who is located within the room with the client and remotely from the clinician, plays a critical role. The client may include both the recipient of the audiological service and in some circumstances local service providers (Figure 3–2). The facilitator and local service providers' roles are considered later in this chapter.

Swanepoel and Hall (2010) have provided a comprehensive critique of peer-reviewed empirical studies using telepractice in

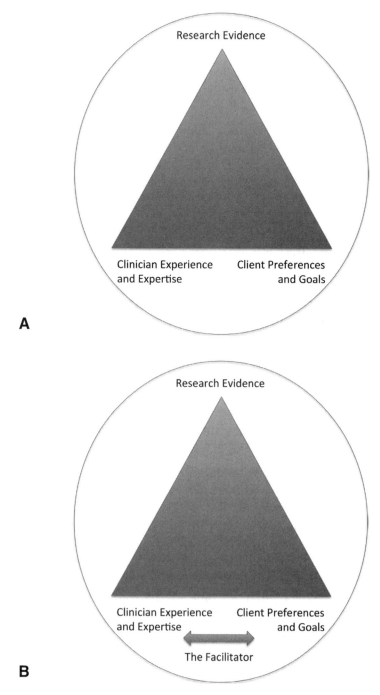

Figure 3–2. A. The principles of evidence-based research. **B.** The principles of evidence-based research adapted for telepractice. From Wong and Hickson (2012). Reprinted with permission of Plural Publishing, Inc.

audiology. The four key areas reviewed included screening, diagnostics, intervention, and patient satisfaction. The review showed that telepractice was utilized most commonly in diagnostics and interventions, with few studies on screening and patient perception. Only a third of the studies had well-designed randomized controls and, according to Wong and Hickson (2012), this is needed to underpin evidence-based practice. Constantinescu and Dornan, in Chapter 10 (this volume), have further examined the importance of evidence-based practice and have defined the levels of evidence required in telepractice. Swanepoel and Hall (2010) found that across these studies, the protocols and service delivery models were often not clear for specific populations, and the understanding of patient and clinician perceptions was poor or incomplete. Further, they found that financial costs and resources for implementing telepractice in audiology within existing health care infrastructures and models were not addressed through systematic investigations and cost analysis. They suggested that future research to gather such evidence requires robust measures to demonstrate reliability and validity of the telepractice models. Therefore, this chapter focuses on evaluation procedures used in broader telepractice to develop frameworks that can be used in future longitudinal evaluations of telepractice models for its application in hearing health care.

Establishing the Need for, the Method, and Limitations of Telepractice

Prior to implementing telepractice, there should be a well-reasoned justification for its use within a specified setting and/or for a specific clinical population. For example, although equal access to health care and educational services is an important consideration for individuals living within rural and remote settings, the availability of appropriate technology, the quality of local Internet connectivity, and the extent to which the identified client population is able to utilize those technologies are also important factors for whether telepractice can or should be implemented.

Within this chapter, we focus on evaluation of the *methods* of telepractice. Methods differ according to the stakeholders involved, the level of their involvement, delivery of the service, and the technology used. Each of these parameters can serve as potential barriers to an efficient and effective service delivery of audiological services through telepractice. Consideration of the continuum of telepractice methodology is necessary to understand the requirements of, and enable optimal engagement of, stakeholders. The role of the stakeholders will vary according to the chosen method of delivery. For example, the locus of responsibility between the clinician and client compared to traditional MOSD may result in the client (and their family) or the facilitator assuming a more autonomous and dominant role in the telepractice model. Therefore, evaluating the efficiencies and effectiveness of telepractice requires a clear understanding of the impact of each of the stakeholder roles to ensure that the dynamics of their relationship and any potential barriers to implementation of telepractice are understood (May, Finch, Mair, & Mort, 2005). Stakeholders' involvement has important implications for the need to develop and evaluate supporting programs (such as training of local service providers) and the inclusion of specific outcome measures, such as the generalizability of skills into the home and broader social environment.

What Are the Different Methods of Telepractice Service Delivery?

Telepractice methods include synchronous interactive telepractice occurring within real time to another clinical site (Figure 3–3A) or to the home (Figure 3–3B), asynchronous (store and forward) to another clinical site, (Figure 3–3C), and telepractice for remote monitoring during self-administered health services either with monitoring (Figure 3–3D) or without monitoring (Figure 3–3E).

Factors influencing the method of service delivery chosen will include the personnel and equipment available and level of intervention provided, such as diagnosis versus rehabilitation (May et al., 2005). More specifically, telepractice to the home and self-administration of services would potentially occur once the client and the facilitator have had training and expertise developed during a clinic-based service delivery model. Access to the technology required also needs to be considered when choos-

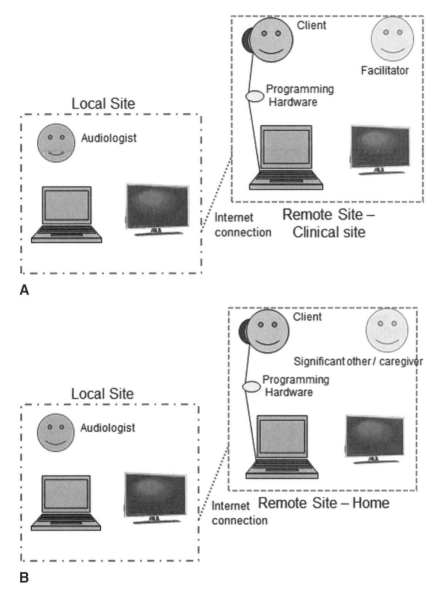

Figure 3–3. Methods of telepractice. **A.** Synchronous interactive to clinical site. **B.** Synchronous interactive to the home. *continues*

ing a telepractice service delivery method, as described earlier. In many cases, these models are used in combination with one another as well as with the more traditional clinic-based services to provide an integrated model of health care.

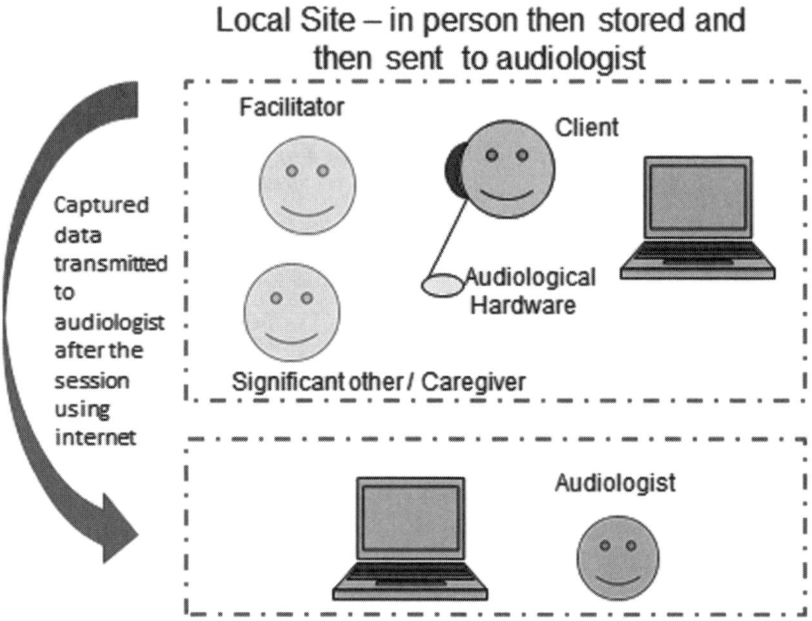

Local Site – in person then stored and then sent to audiologist

Facilitator

Client

Captured data transmitted to audiologist after the session using internet

Audiological Hardware

Significant other / Caregiver

Audiologist

C

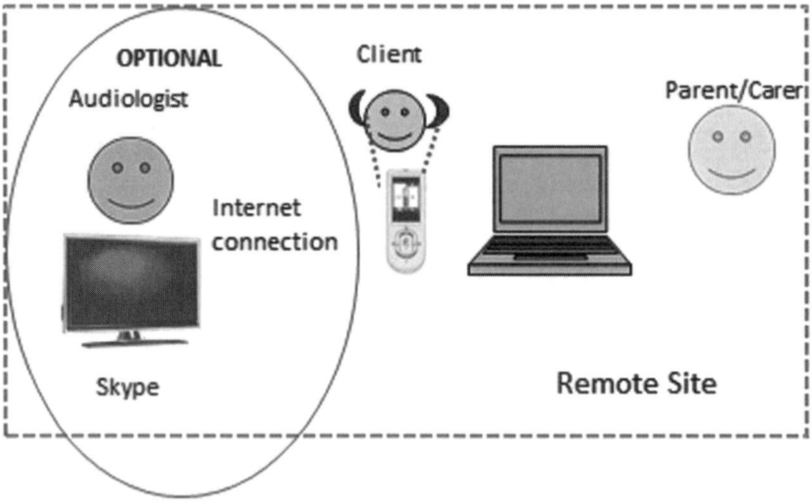

OPTIONAL

Audiologist

Client

Parent/Carer

Internet connection

Skype

Remote Site

D

Figure 3–3. *continued* **C.** Asynchronous. **D.** Remote monitoring: non-interactive. *continues*

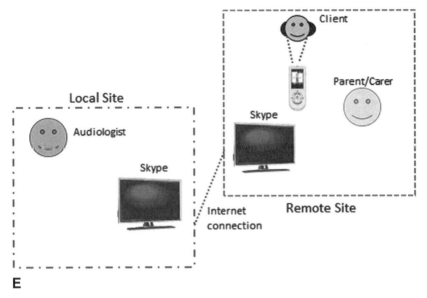

Figure 3–3. *continued* **E.** Remote monitoring: interactive.

Table 3–1 outlines the stakeholder involvement for the various telepractice methods used within the various models of telepractice service delivery. Synchronous telepractice to another clinical site is the most common model used and typically includes the clinician, the client, and a facilitator (often a clinician or health care worker from a related discipline). The clinician has a moderate level of involvement, directing the session and instructing the facilitator to ensure efficient and effective delivery of the session.

Telepractice to the home is an emerging model involving caregivers or significant others as the key to facilitators of the audiological session. This model requires greater involvement from the family, which, through empowerment of these stakeholders, maximizes the opportunities for integration of skills into daily life. This model benefits individuals in more remote areas as well as those who are less mobile and/or time poor and unable to attend clinic-based sessions. A fundamental consideration of the stakeholders in this model is that the parent, significant other, or caregiver would need to adopt a hybrid role of the "coach" or "facilitator" as well as their standard role within the relationship with the client, as a family member, for example

Table 3–1. Telepractice Continuum and the Impact on Stakeholder Relationships

Telepractice	Clinician	Client/Family	Facilitator (e.g., another clinician or family member)
Synchronous interactive (e.g., telemapping to another clinical site with the facilitator and the client or to the home with just the client/family member)	Directs the stakeholder involvement	Dependent on the clinician via the facilitator	Facilitates the clinicians instructions
Asynchronous (e.g., otoscopy images being captured by the facilitator and stored on a computer or a digital storage device before being forwarded to the clinician)	Dependent on results obtained by the facilitator. Decision making based on the data collected by the facilitator	Dependent on the facilitator	Directs the client involvement
Remote monitoring—noninteractive (e.g., auditory training programs downloaded onto a computer or digital source or from a commercial website)	May be involved in monitoring and feedback	Independently administered	May not be involved/optional role
Remote monitoring—interactive (e.g., m-health; uploading of client information; e.g., a client is able to perform basic mapping of his or her cochlear implant independent of the clinician using remote assistant fitting of cochlear implants [RAFI] (Botros et al., 2013).This is monitored by the clinician either synchronously or asynchronously.	Monitoring and provision of feedback/future directions	Independently administered; future direction based on feedback of clinician	May not be involved/optional role

(Robins et al., 2005). This coaching role would be embedded in the model to also facilitate language development and communication. The use of telepractice to deliver asynchronous health services (where the clinician may not be present during the session but may monitor the outcomes over time) provides the opportunity for clients and significant others or caregivers to facilitate their own sessions and develop autonomy in managing their own health.

The synchronous interactive model of telepractice, facilitated by another clinician on the remote end, is often limited to one or two episodes of service that focus on diagnostics or screening (Swanepoel & Hall, 2010). Implementation of longitudinal models of telepractice in audiology is currently under investigation, particularly in the field of cochlear implantation when clients require ongoing audiological support over a lifetime. Krupinski et al. (2011) describe evidence of longitudinal telepractice models in other health service delivery programs. Specifically, otolaryngology services provided by the Arizona Telemedicine Program, established in 1997, and the Baycrest Telehealth program, developed in 2005, demonstrate the principles of a successful telepractice program. Training and education of staff and facilitators, careful evaluation and assessment of procedures and outcomes, and flexibility within the infrastructure (to ensure the telepractice model was the most appropriate model for stakeholders) were considered critical to the success of long-term applications. In each of these cases, ongoing evaluation of the models used provided the evidence base to ensure the sustainability and development of these programs. In the future, evidence-based practice will guide the identification of the appropriate model of service delivery, including the type of telepractice model best suited for integrated service delivery and client management.

Stakeholder Influence in Telepractice

Evaluating the development and implementation of telepractice should account for characteristics of all stakeholders, such as attitude, age, training level, motivation, and culture, and additional considerations for the client (and facilitator), such as level of cognition or presence of additional disabilities.

Attitude

Clark and Goodwin (2011) identified the importance of attitude of stakeholders. They found that adoption of telepractice models can be hindered by organizations and clinicians who have difficulty adjusting to the methods of delivery and the resulting organizational changes. This, in turn, reduces the demand with the potential client market. Leadership culture and organization infrastructure that fail to support the innovation of a telepractice model are among one of the major barriers to widespread use of telepractice in health care. Alkmim et al. (2012) also found that attitudes of stakeholders such as health managers, clinicians, and clients were pivotal in the implementation of successful telepractice programs. They recommended the implementation of training programs to desensitize the use of new approaches and to provide all stakeholders with the opportunity to develop an effective working relationship.

Age

Age is often linked with attitude toward technology (Morris & Venkatesh, 2000). Singh (2014) conducted a series of studies investigating attitudes of stakeholders, including clinicians, clients, and facilitators (in this case, family members). He showed that the age of the client influences the clinician's attitude to using telepractice, with all practitioners indicating a willingness to use this model for clients aged 13 to 65 years. However, there was less support among clinicians for using telepractice with younger or older clients. Yet, when Singh (2014) evaluated the willingness of 224 clients who had recently received audiological services to consider telepractice for their future access to audiology, 75% of the respondents indicated a moderate to extreme willingness to have a telepractice model (Figure 3–4). Respondents to the survey were on average 67 years of age. Clearly, there was a mismatch in the assumption of clinicians

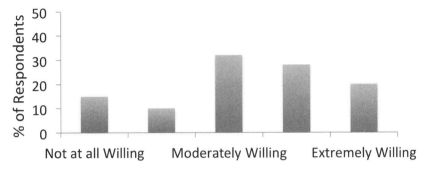

Figure 3–4. Patient willingness to use teleaudiology. From Singh (2014). Reprinted with permission of Gurjit Singh.

who disregarded the use of telepractice with people over 65, when in fact, that particular age group was willing to experience that method of service delivery.

Mitchell, Rhodes, and Grossman (2004) demonstrated the effectiveness of telepractice in management of long-term care residents in a nursing home who required a wide range of specialty medical services. Fifty-five percent of the elderly residents were satisfied with the telepractice model compared to 40% satisfaction with the in-person consultation. The remaining 5% of residents had no preference. Telepractice would appear to be a viable model irrespective of the client's age. Psarros, van Wanrooy, and Pascoe (2012) found that it was possible to perform cochlear implant mapping using telepractice with five cochlear implant recipients aged over 65 years. However, the effectiveness and efficiency was variable. That is, the time taken to deliver the cochlear implant mapping session was longer than that taken for younger adults and for children without additional physical, medical, or communication needs. The satisfaction ratings were variable, with two of the five clients citing dissatisfaction with the quality of the videoconferencing, that they would prefer a within-clinic model. Although this would not necessarily exclude this age group from inclusion in a telepractice method, individual circumstances would need to be evaluated to ascertain the suitability of this method for particular clients. The impact of age of stakeholders on telepractice, although a consideration, appears to be attitudinal and is predominantly impacted by motivation and willingness, and hence is not a single influencing factor in the implementation of a telepractice model.

Motivation and Willingness

It is the consumer experience that will drive the future of telepractice. If consumers are provided with accurate and relevant information, it is possible that they will try telepractice, and it will be the quality of their experience that will qualify their perceptions and lead to a reengagement with and/or an ultimate preference for a telepractice model. Victoor, Delnoij, Friel, and Rademaker (2012) found that although patients use comparative information in deciding which model of medical service to select, the level of understanding of such material might be limited due to low levels of health literacy. The two aspects of health literacy—an individual's health literacy and the health literacy environment—can affect the motivation and willingness to use telepractice.

An individual's health literacy is his or her knowledge, motivation, and competencies to understand and apply health information. The health literacy environment is "the infrastructure, policies, processes, materials and relationships that exist within the health system that make it easier or more difficult for consumers to navigate, understand and use health information and services to make effective decisions about health and healthcare and take appropriate action" (Australian Commission on Safety and Quality in Health Care [ACSQHC], 2013, p. 5). Both of these aspects of health literacy have the potential to provide consumers with the necessary information to choose telepractice as a model of service delivery.

One of the main motivators for choice of a service is access. The majority of consumers want a service close to home, with easy access to transportation and available parking at the site of their clinical service provider. Nevertheless, Victoor et al. (2012) found those who were highly educated with larger incomes were more willing to travel to get their services. These findings suggest that one cannot assume that recipients of services who potentially could benefit from telepractice will want to use it as it may be viewed as inferior in quality to a face-to face practice. It is important to note that the choice of the service is an intricate interaction between personal and provider characteristics such as the development of trust. Positive experiences with a particular model and social influence, such as reports from other recipients of the service, can develop the trust in the service methodology, which may impact the client's decision making. If service providers want to increase the uptake of telepractice services, they need to carefully consider the information they provide and how they deliver it to the consumer.

Cognition

ASHA guidelines recommend consideration of the level of cognitive functioning of a client when using telepractice. The effectiveness of telepractice could be impacted by the cognitive, behavioral, and motivational characteristics and the ability to maintain attention (ASHA, n.d.)). The influence of cognition on the effectiveness of a telepractice model has not been formally evaluated in the literature. Sato, Clifford, Silverman, and Davies (2009) suggested that the required level of cognitive sophistication could be a barrier to the effectiveness of telepractice with children and adolescents. They suggested that an adolescent who is not motivated to participate could render a telepractice session ineffective through not communicating clearly. It is difficult to determine whether this "poor motivation" was due to cognitive sophistication or their capacity to participate. However, Kopel, Nunn, and Dossetor (2001) found that a telepsychiatry program with children and adolescents using telepractice had 97% satisfaction ratings from the recipients of the program.

Additional Considerations

Children and adults with additional needs such as vision impairment, autism, cerebral palsy, and cognitive delay were included in a feasibility study of cochlear implant programming using telepractice (Psarros et al., 2012). Although all sessions with this population were able to be completed, the average times taken for these sessions compared with sessions of clients who did not have additional needs were longer (Figure 3–5).

The average telepractice session time was 28 minutes for cochlear implant recipients without additional needs, 38 minutes for those with additional needs (such as cerebral palsy and developmental delay), and 45 minutes for elderly cochlear implant recipients. This was not unexpected as clients with complex needs routinely require longer sessions for their management in face-to-face clinical sessions. Therefore, although age and additional disabilities have not been studied in detail, these factors and their interaction with the role of the remote facilitator of telepractice are important considerations. Psarros et al. (2012) found that with younger participants and those with additional needs, the facilitator had a more active role than with other recipient groups. Greater involvement was required on the part of the facilitator to ensure that clients were aware of what was required and keep them on task. However, they noted that the level of engagement was consistent with what would be required for a within-clinic model of service delivery.

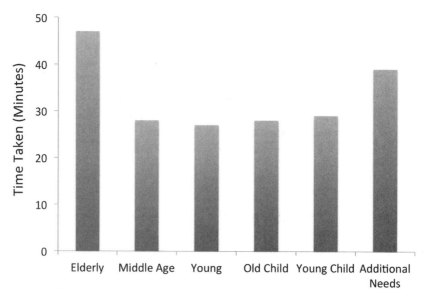

Figure 3–5. Time taken for populations during cochlear implant mapping. Based on Psarros, van Wanrooy, and Pascoe (2012).

Effectiveness of Telepractice Models— Clinical Outcomes and Quality of Service

Evaluating the equivalency in clinical outcomes and quality of outcomes with telepractice may not always capture alternative or additional outcomes that may result. Effectiveness is used instead of equivalency in our model for evaluation, providing the capacity to evaluate equivalency while also capturing additional features that a telepractice model may provide over other MOSD.

Clinical Outcomes

Clinical equivalency has underpinned most telepractice research. A series of studies on clinical application of telepractice at the University of Queensland has evaluated the diagnostic accuracy, therapeutic outcomes, and clinical, therapeutic, and societal efficacy (Figure 3–6). Emphasis on equivalency of service delivery

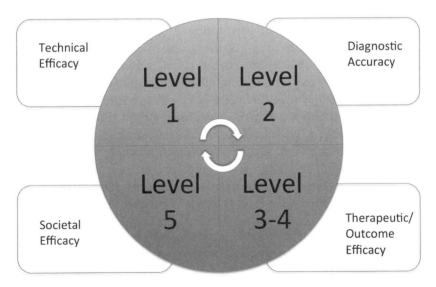

Figure 3–6. Broad experience and research across five domains of telerehabilitation research. Adapted from Fryback and Thornbury (1991), by Trevor Russell (unpublished) at the Telerehabilitation Research Unit, School of Health and Rehabilitation Sciences, The University of Queensland.

using telepractice for physiotherapy, speech-language pathology, and audiology with the eHAB telerehabilitation videoconferencing (VC) system has been widely reported based on this model (Constantinescu et al., 2010; Rushbrooke, 2012; Russell, Buttrum, Wootton, & Jull, 2003; Waite, Cahill, Theodoros, Busuttin, & Russell, 2006). These studies have evaluated equivalency in clinical performance and outcomes of clients on tasks specific to their treatment, time taken to deliver the service, and effectiveness measures that are discussed later in this chapter.

Rushbrooke (2012) established the validity of cochlear implant mapping using telepractice through demonstrating equivalency in outcomes compared to a within-clinic model of service delivery. There were no significant differences measured in the electrical current levels obtained for cochlear implant electrodes measured across both within the clinic or when using telepractice. Further, there were no significant differences in speech perception performance as measured with sentence and word-level testing in younger cochlear implant recipients aged between 5 and 22 years.

Effectiveness of the telepractice model can be readily measured against existing quality standards for a particular service. For example, Martin and Raine's (2013) published quality standards for cochlear implant service delivery can be used as a "checklist" to ensure that all aspects of the service have been addressed. Minimum requirements for the stakeholders, resources, and processes necessary for cochlear implant service delivery are listed. The checklist describes a framework of evaluation for effectiveness of a service irrespective of the model of service delivery used. Failure to meet the minimum requirements of quality standards would suggest that effectiveness in the standard of the service delivered has not been met.

Quality of Outcomes

Evaluating the qualitative effectiveness of telepractice has predominantly used satisfaction questionnaires (Eikelboom et al., 2014; Kopel et al., 2001; Rushbrooke, 2012; Wesarg et al., 2010) and/or interviews (Dally & Conway, 2008). Variables including the technology, location of service delivery, and the stakeholders involved will impact the quality of telepractice sessions. It is expected that most stakeholders have had a within-clinic experience that could function as a reference point prior to initiating telepractice. Satisfaction questionnaires could be used to determine the baseline of experience of the stakeholder with each model of service delivery. Dally and Conway (2008) reviewed outcomes and effectiveness of a telepractice program delivering early intervention to children with hearing and/or vision loss over 1 year. Experimental design included the use of structured interviews and questionnaires presented prior to service delivery and 12 months later. Qualitative questionnaires that investigated expectations of the service were given to all stakeholders, including clinicians and the recipients of the service. The recipients included the families of children with vision and hearing loss, as well as local service providers such as teachers and speech-language pathologists. The level of experience of stakeholders was a question asked as part of their survey. Comparative analysis was performed between the responses from the questionnaires, client interviews, and some best practice service delivery examples identified in the literature.

The assessment intervals and content areas of questionnaires and interviews, based on the literature and the authors' model of evaluation proposed in Figure 3–1, can be found in Table 3–2. The multifaceted nature of questions provides the framework for identifying the effectiveness and efficiencies and how these are impacted by the stakeholder engagement while controlling for the individual characteristics of stakeholders identified earlier.

Parameters outlined in Table 3–2 provide the framework for designing an evaluation of telepractice, advocating a mixed-methods approach of questionnaire and interview. For example, if evaluating the effectiveness of telepractice in cochlear implant mapping, evaluation points recommended would be prior to implementation and at various intervals postimplementation and should include all of the stakeholders, with clear definition of their characteristics such as age, previous training, and motivation.

Table 3–2. Variables and Questions to Include in Questionnaire and Interview Development for Evaluating Telepractice

Telepractice type	Synchronous to clinic
	Synchronous to home
	Asynchronous
	Remote monitoring—noninteractive
	Remote monitoring—interactive
Stakeholder (separate interview/ questionnaire for each) (Clinician Client Facilitator)	Age (group) 0–11; 12–20; 21–30; 31–40; 41–50; 51–60; 61–70; 71–80; 81–90; 91–100
	Considerations: (Specify) cognition, additional needs
	Motivation: (Rate: 1 = not motivated to 5 = highly motivated)
Interval of questionnaire/ interview	Prior to telepractice
	Immediately following the session
	Short term (e.g., 1 month) after
	Long term (chronic care) ongoing (after 12 months)
Technology	How much training/information did you have before this service?[1]
	How much has the technology changed since you first delivered/received telepractice?[3]
	How much has the procedure changed since you first delivered/received telepractice?[3]
Efficiencies	QUESTIONNAIRE RATING
	How efficient was this service?[3]
	How timely was the service delivered?[3]
	How easy was it to deliver/receive this service?[1,3]
	How anxious were you with this procedure?[2]
	How did you feel about the procedure?[2]
	How easy was the access to the service?[3]

Table 3–2. *continued*

Effectiveness	QUESTIONNAIRE RATING
	How effective was this service?[3]
	Would you use this service again?[3]
	How comfortable were you with delivering/receiving this service?[2]
	How was the sound quality?[3]
	How was the visual quality?[3]
	How did the telepractice equipment impact the delivery/receipt of your service?[2,3]
	INTERVIEW QUESTIONS
	How could this service be more effective?[1,2,3]
	How would you view this service in the short term/long term?[3]
	How would you describe the interaction with all the participants in the service?[1,2]
Additional factors	Describe any additional knowledge or skills you have developed from using telepractice.[1,2]
	How would you describe the roles of the people involved in the service delivery?[2]
	How does this impact your service in the short term/long term?[1,2,3]

Note. Questions relating to human,[1] social,[2] and institutional[3] capital for identifying sustainability as indicated.

Source: Based on Rogers (2006).

Efficiencies of a Telepractice Model

Timeliness of service delivery, cost-effectiveness, satisfaction of stakeholders, ease of implementation, and access to services are commonly reported areas reflecting the efficacy of the service and will be considered when evaluating efficiencies of telepractice.

Stakeholder Satisfaction

Questionnaires or surveys of patient satisfaction are common tools for measuring effectiveness of health care irrespective of the model of service delivery (Kopel et al., 2001). These can be impacted by stakeholder characteristics, level of the response rate, workload of participants (prioritization of tasks), the time interval of when the questionnaire was completed prior to or following the service, and literacy levels. Kopel et al. (2001) reported the satisfaction ratings of all stakeholders, including clinicians, clients, and facilitators, using telepractice to deliver mental health services to children and adolescents. Overall, each group of stakeholders reported high satisfaction ratings in areas relating to service and technology. However, the authors had a 60% response rate from the clients and a 74% response rate from the facilitators. Data collection was impacted by the heavy workload on the facilitators who were local service providers, who found completion of such surveys a burden. A more effective means of data collection, including a quick online questionnaire at the end of the session, could possibly have circumvented this issue.

Bakken et al. (2006) validated the readability of Telemedicine Satisfaction and Use Questionnaire (TSUQ) (in both English and Spanish) used to provide perceptions of usefulness and actual utilization of telemedicine as having a readability at an eighth-grade level using Flesch-Kinkaid ratings. This level of literacy would preclude completion by almost 60% of Australians who were identified as having low levels of health literacy (ACSQHC, 2013). As addressed earlier, health literacy impacts the level of training. This, in turn, can impact the accuracy of the evaluation tools used, requiring careful attention to ensure that clients and facilitators have the opportunity to provide accurate feedback, which may require an interview rather than completion of a written questionnaire (ACSQHC, 2013). Interviewing with open-ended questions was used by Dally and Conway (2008) and Singh (2014) to evaluate the efficiencies of telepractice.

Emotional reactions to telepractice were identified by Kopel et al. (2001), who found that a small proportion of parents and children (3%) reported feelings of self-consciousness, embarrassment, and slight anxiety when receiving mental health services delivered by telepractice. Further, the same proportion of participants felt that the equipment used for telepractice interfered with their consultation. In the same study, which had rural clinicians present as facilitators during the sessions with young children or adolescents and their caregivers during mental health consultations, 3% of facilitators experienced self-consciousness, slight anxiety, and embarrassment, with 13% perceiving that telepractice interfered with the consultation. The discrepancy between the facilitators and the client and caregiver perceptions of the impact of the equipment, highlights the importance of considering all stakeholders in the evaluation of telepractice.

To date, there have been no published data for the satisfaction ratings from the facilitators of telepractice in audiology. The exact role and the level of training needed by the facilitator is an area that requires further investigation. Unpublished data from a feasibility study conducted by Psarros et al. (2012) found that the facilitators, who were predominantly hearing health care professionals other than audiologists, were generally satisfied with the use of telepractice when they facilitated remote cochlear implant mapping sessions for recipients aged between 12 months and 82 years. Facilitator satisfaction was good to excellent overall (Figure 3–7), consistent with the clinician (audiologists) ratings. Recipient ratings were not as favorable but on average were still rated as good satisfaction.

Telepractice and audiology rely heavily on use of instrumentation and assistive technologies, and those involved in receiving and delivering services may already have skills and knowledge to generalize to telepractice technologies. However, the literature suggests that this does not seem to influence a client's decision to partake in telepractice. Bakken et al. (2006) found education level and computer literacy were not significant when assessing client satisfaction with telepractice.

The time interval for evaluating telepractice has been highlighted by Whitten and Love (2005), who caution that there could be bias in questionnaires caused by their administration immediately after a service when there is a short-term positive impression and the fact that, particularly in the case of rural residents, they are being offered a service they may not otherwise be able to access. However, Bakken et al. (2006) found that satisfaction ratings of urban recipients were higher than those of rural

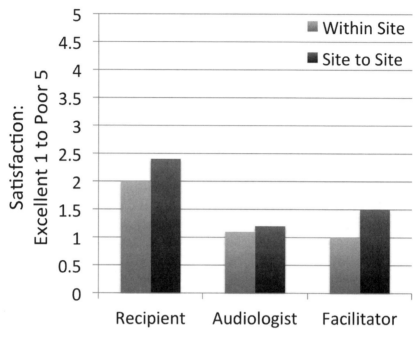

Figure 3–7. Stakeholder (clinician, recipient, and facilitator) satisfaction ratings for telepractice in cochlear implant mapping sessions, with 1 = excellent satisfaction to 5 = poor satisfaction. Based on Psarros, van Wanrooy, and Pascoe (2012).

recipients of telemedicine. Yet, they attribute this partly due to the fact that the urban population were interviewed in person, whereas the rural population completed written surveys.

A mixed-methods approach of evaluation combining direct interview and survey was used by Singh (2014) to investigate the attitudes of the stakeholders in telepractice, including audiologists, and recipients in a series of three studies. A qualitative study interviewed 11 hearing health care professionals and identified their perceived advantages and disadvantages. Accessibility and convenience was identified as the major advantage, but the perceived disadvantage noted by the clinicians was that it could negatively impact the relationship with the recipient of the service. Singh (2014) surveyed a larger group of 202 professionals working in private practice (109), not for profit (53), or their own practice (28). Overall, a large proportion of the clinicians had a negative attitude toward telepractice, and although they acknowledged potential benefits in accessibility, they did not anticipate any effect on hearing health care. The impact of age of the recipient on the attitudes of the clinicians was investigated in a further survey, which evaluated perceptions of the willingness to use telepractice with pediatric versus adult clients. Fifty-five clinicians primarily worked with children and 126 with adults.

In summary, satisfaction and perception ratings of stakeholders can be impacted by the method of data collection. A combination of interview and survey of all stakeholders is recommended at an interval immediately after the service delivery and potentially after longitudinal use of the telepractice procedure, once the stakeholders have had greater experience with this model of service delivery.

Ease of Implementation

Clinical application of telepractice requires attention to clinicians and the clinical processes (Tang et al., 2007). Lack of knowledge of implementation of telepractice has been identified as one the major barriers of implementation throughout the world (WHO, 2011). Some clinicians may take some time before they feel comfortable using telepractice and may need a period of acclimatization (Wesarg et al., 2010). Wesarg et al. (2010) found that most clinicians found it easy and safe to use telepractice for cochlear implant fittings but found that it increased the time taken to complete all aspects of the service delivered within the session. A recent study by Eikelboom et al. (2014) evaluated the recipient and clinician's experiences with telepractice and found statistically significant agreement in the ratings that were given for the voice quality, video quality, and overall experience for both groups.

WHO recommends information communication and technology (ICT) training be provided to all health care professionals to familiarize them with telepractice platforms (WHO, 2010). Tools used to provide telepractice should be readily available to ensure ready adoption into clinical practice. For a clinical model incorporating telepractice to be successful, it needs to be sustainable. That is, once its validity has been shown, it must be adopted into everyday practice and continue to function with high activity levels (Zanaboni & Wootton, 2012). There are two stages needed for technology to be adopted:

1. The individual or organization must become acquainted with the technology under consideration.
2. A favorable or unfavorable opinion about the technology needs to be determined—that is, the advantages and disadvantages of the technology need to be clarified.

In clinical practice, the adoption of certain techniques and procedures—and technologies—goes through a series of stages, and key to its success is that it is easy to use, time efficient, and readily integrated. Stakeholder "buy-in" at an organizational, clinical, client, and facilitator level is pivotal in this process (Figure 3–8).

In scoping or researching telepractice as a viable option of service, delivery barriers and facilitators to adopting the models must be identified and used to develop guidelines for the implementation of the practice. When considering the benefits of a telepractice model, its integration into clinical practice extends beyond conducting validation research. Ease of implementation requires risk and sustainability analyses of telepractice, including privacy and security issues. Each country has its own security standards, and when conducting telepractice across borders, it is critical that regulations are considered. Watzlaf, Fahima, Moeini, and Firouzan (2010) conducted a risk analysis that reviewed potential breaches of confidentiality and privacy, integrity issues, and availability of service when conducting telepractice for rehabilitation. Careful consideration of their guidelines that incorporate appropriate consenting between parties, regular auditing of processes, and training in procedures as technological changes

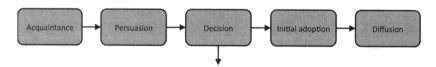

Figure 3–8. Stages in the adoption of technology. Based on Zanaboni and Wootton (2012).

occur could provide effective sustainability and implementation of the telepractice model. With continuous evolution of the tools used in telepractice, ongoing research and data collection must account for the fact that the applications and technology used are in a constant state of development (Bashshur & Shannon, 2009). The dynamic nature of the technology and applications can have a positive impact in that costs continue to decrease with technological innovation, increased competition deregulation, and wider use of wireless transmission methods (Cameron et al., 1998).

Cost-Effectiveness

Cost-effectiveness was identified as one of the major barriers to the adoption to mHealth initiatives around the world, which was exacerbated by competing health priorities (WHO, 2011). The acceptance of telepractice will occur when there is either no change to or an improvement in outcomes, with a reduction of or no change in financial cost. Table 3–3 illustrates a model based on a model proposed by Ruckdaschel et al. (2006) comparing quality, costs, and the impact of telepractice.

Financial decision makers are usually interested in a break-even analysis in that revenue should equal or surpass all costs. This framework in Table 3–3 can evaluate whether the telepractice is cost neutral, more costly, or more cost-effective in relation to the outcomes in equivalency of the quality of services provided using alternative models of service delivery.

Policy makers focus on clinical efficacy and cost-effectiveness; however, most telepractice services are not mature enough for the true economic potential analysis to be conducted. Financial concerns about cost efficiency coupled with limited documentation of clinical outcomes have restrained the expansion and use of telepractice (Cameron et al., 1998). One solution is for policy makers to align their organization with government or nongovernment sectors that deliver telepractice to maximize affordability and sustainability (WHO, 2010). Regardless, one of the simplest areas to report on cost-effectiveness is time and travel. Brown-Connelly (2002) evaluated the travel information from 741 patients receiving 27 different specialist interventions

Table 3–3. Qualitative and Quantitative Evaluation Telepractice

Comparing Costs	Comparing Quality		
	Impaired With Telepractice	No Change With Telepractice	Improved With Telepractice
Declined with telepractice	Impaired quality in face of savings	Acceptance of telepractice measures	Acceptance of telepractice measures
No change with telepractice	Rejection of telepractice	Decision based on political and societal preferences	Acceptance of telepractice measures
Increased with telepractice	Rejection of telepractice	Rejection of telepractice measures	Improvement in quality accepted as being "worth the cost"

Source: Based on Ruckdaschel et al. (2006).

with telepractice. They found the telepractice model reduced travel distance by an average of 170 km, with an average saving of 130 minutes, having implications for the timeliness of the service delivery.

Cost-effectiveness of a telepractice model for delivering cochlear implant services was reported to include up to $200,000 of savings per year compared to clinicians traveling to regional and remote areas to deliver clinical services (Griffith, 2012). The savings factored in the costs of room hire, travel costs (including flights, car travel, clinician time), and accommodation costs, compared with the investment in technology required for delivering telepractice. The equipment used for telepractice was standard "off-the-shelf" technology, which was commercially available and used for purposes other than service delivery (e.g., videoconferencing for meetings and supporting of clinicians in remote regions). This is consistent with WHO (2010) recommendations for facilitating the cost-effectiveness of telepractice.

Cost-effectiveness needs to include the costs of capital expenditure as well as the personal costs and stakeholder costs involved in the telepractice, which can be difficult to measure. Identification of indirect costs and benefits of the human, social, and organization capital can provide evidence for sustainability of telepractice (Rogers, 2006). Rogers (2006) highlights the importance of evaluating the impact of human, social, and institutional capital—that is,

- Human capital—skills and knowledge
- Social capital—support networks, based on trust and reciprocity
- Institutional capital—based on processes, systems, and products that continue to be used after a project ends

Earlier in Table 3–2, we identified a framework for evaluating telepractice that has embedded questions that can elicit this information. Dally and Conway (2008) emphasized the need for a longitudinal evaluation to identify the sustainability of the processes, networks, and systems of telepractice. As indicated in Table 3–2, evaluation should not be just performed at one interval; it should be performed longitudinally to provide information about sustainability of the model.

Specific indirect costs and benefits that have been identified by the authors can be found in Table 3–4, which identifies stakeholder costs and benefits identified through implementation of this evaluation process.

Direct costs such as purchasing of equipment for telepractice are balanced with direct benefits such as savings on travel for the client, whereas indirect costs such as training time needed to enable facilitator involvement are balanced with indirect benefits such as the ability to cross-pollinate skills and provide opportunities for training and generalization into the local environment.

Access and Timeliness of Service Delivery

Choosing when, where, and how to seek health care is a complex process and influenced by many factors, particularly within the current consumer-driven market. Motivation to choose an

Table 3–4. Costs and Benefits (Direct and Indirect) for Stakeholders for Telepractice

Cost/Benefit	Stakeholder—Client	Organization—Clinician	Stakeholder—Facilitator
COST	Equipment for telepractice if home based Internet if home based	Equipment for telepractice (e.g., Internet) and technology Room hire (if to other site) Training time required for facilitator/stakeholders Salary of facilitator Lack of reimbursement	Training time needed
BENEFIT	Access to service Reduced travel time Reduced costs for travel Reduced impact on work/education /family Reduced stress (travel time and less disruption to work and education) Quicker access to troubleshooting Generalization of skills learnt into local environment	No outreach travel costs Utilization of existing resources Integration of existing technology Quicker delivery of troubleshooting Facilitate generalization of skills into the home environment Flexibility of service provision Ease of scheduling Training of local service providers Training of new staff in other sites Professional development of facilitator	Reduced stress of recipient and family Professional development— new skill development Deeper insight into procedures as they are adapted to delivery and receipt of telepractice

audiological telepractice appointment includes improved access to specialists, whereas other factors such as flexibility in appointment times, meeting with a practitioner in an emergency, reducing waiting room time, and obtaining quicker appointments stimulated some motivation but were less likely to motivate the decision to use telepractice (Singh, 2014) (Figure 3–9).

Factors least likely to motivate a telepractice appointment were the concern that the audiologists could not perform an examination of the client or that they could not perform their examination of the hearing device. Lack of social contact, being in the same room, change in eye contact, and the bond with the practitioner did not impact the decision to use telepractice (Figure 3–10).

A similar survey of 450 parents (mean age of 31.4 years) of children with hearing loss (mean age of 6.3 years) revealed that 90% were moderately to extremely willing to have a telepractice

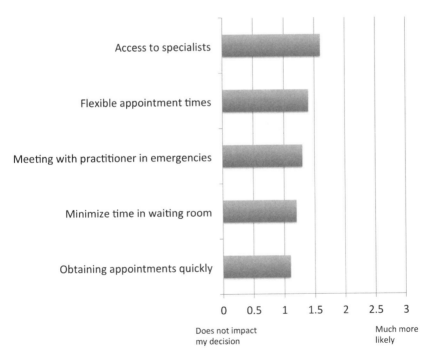

Figure 3–9. Factors most likely to motivate a telepractice appointment. From Singh (2014). Reprinted with permission of Gurjit Singh.

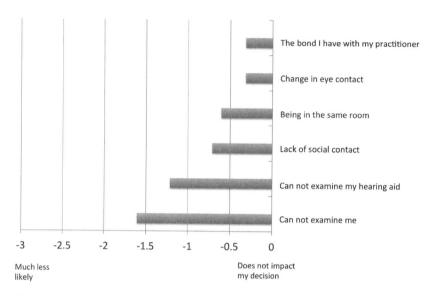

Figure 3–10. Factors least likely to motivate a telepractice appointment. From Singh (2014). Reprinted with permission of Gurjit Singh.

model of audiological service. This is at odds with the clinician survey, which indicated that telepractice would be best suited for clients between 13 and 65 years of age, reinforcing the need for clinicians to be more consultative when considering MOSD and ensuring they are capturing the clients' needs. Absences from school, stress of travel, and time taken from employment are commonly cited reasons that parents would prefer a telepractice model for delivery of health care for their child (Sato et al., 2009). Research conducted in the United States on families of young children with a hearing impairment, prior to the implementation of telepractice programs for this population, showed that 28% of families moved residence to be within closer proximity to hearing health care services (Calderon, Bargones, & Sidmon, 1998). It is important to recognize that this decision is a significant life change and may not be an option for all families. Employment and proximity to family and friend support are key factors that influence a family's decision to relocate to access services, which may not be necessary if a telepractice model of service delivery were available.

Yet, Whitten and Love (2005) found clients might not necessarily choose to use a telepractice model even if they did have to travel to access services. The decision to travel for services was based on a perception that services provided in major centers might be superior to those presented in regional and remote areas. Bakken et al. (2006) found good acceptance of telepractice irrespective of whether they were urban and rural clients, which further highlights that decisions to provide or access services are not based entirely on geography.

Young and Ireson (2003) reported use of telepractice contributed to clinician confidence in the effectiveness of delivering a service in a timely manner. Specifically, clinicians favorably rated the speed at which a diagnosis could be made and a treatment could be ordered, showing high agreement with the effectiveness of telepractice.

Implicit Aspects of Telepractice

Evaluating the effectiveness and efficiencies of telepractice may reveal implicit aspects that can impact its choice as a model of service delivery. The stakeholders involved in telepractice have a unique opportunity to develop and in turn generalize the skills shared throughout the session. The impact of telepractice on the stress and lifestyle of the stakeholders is an additional variable that is often reported but has not been formally researched or reported in the literature. In keeping with this, there is potential for telepractice to mitigate the "third-party disability" that is often identified in family members of someone with a hearing loss, who may experience limitations in activity and restrictions in participation (Scarinci, Worrall, & Hickson, 2012). Finally, the strategic positioning of an organization that offers a telepractice model is emerging as having strong commercial and social impact.

Generalization of Skills

Telepractice is an opportunity to extend and develop the skill set of local service providers and family members or significant others who may be involved in the service delivery as facilitators. An evaluation of the RIDBC teleschool program found that local service providers who provided in-person services to the children and their families in their local settings were able to apply and adapt their skill set to include specialized skills learned from the telepractice provider (Dally & Conway, 2008).

Telepractice into the home may provide yet unquantifiable but qualitative benefits, including the generalization of skills and the ability of the service provider (clinician) to observe the client (and other family members) in his or her natural environment. This provides great insight for designing appropriate intervention that targets the needs of the client and his or her significant others, resulting in sessions tailored to being more relevant and meaningful to all the stakeholders (Sato et al., 2009).

Impact on Stakeholders Confidence and Well-Being

The use of telepractice in the early intervention of hearing- and vision-impaired children resulted in families feeling empowered and supported, with a reduction in stress and anxiety levels (Dally & Conway, 2008). Sarant and Garrard (2014) reported that parents of children with hearing loss, in particular with cochlear implants and language delay, have higher levels of stress than the normative population. The stress as measured on the Parenting Stress Index (Abidin, 1995) was identified to result from time demands, discipline, and concerns for their child's future, requiring support and intervention.

Young and Ireson (2003) evaluated the confidence in decision making of clinicians when using telepractice to deliver clinical services to children in a school setting in both rural and urban areas. Prior to commencing the service, clinicians initially expressed their concerns about the effectiveness of telepractice for diagnosing and treating the children and for interacting with the family or caregivers. Following the session, satisfaction questionnaires reflected a high level of confidence.

Eckberg, Meyer, Scarinci, Grenness, and Hickson (2012) identified active engagement of family members in audiological appointments as a means of mitigating the third-party disability that can result from having a family member with a hearing loss. Family members can be a key stakeholder in facilitating the telepractice process. Although research on family member involvement in audiology is just emerging, literature in other areas of rehabilitation, such as speech-language pathology, has shown that this family-centered care leads to better outcomes, reinforcing the use of family members in the facilitation of telepractice.

Organizational Factors

Telepractice provides an organization with the opportunity to train new staff in other sites (Hughes et al., 2012), ease of scheduling, and stakeholder confidence (Dally & Conway, 2007; Young & Ireson, 2003). Involvement with local service providers and clients in rural and remote regions and in urban areas provides an organization with the opportunity to demonstrate the range of service models they provide and in turn stimulate a broader market for their services. The development of the WHO International Classification of Function (ICF) in 2001 for hearing has resulted in a shift from impairment, or hearing loss, to include activity and participation, providing a more holistic approach to the client. Speech and language therapists have found that there is now a more flexible choice of the model of service delivery used moving away from the traditional medical model (Wylie, McAllister, Davidson, & Marshall, 2013). Audiology Australia's (2014) position paper incorporates the ICF brief core sets and identifies how they can be integrated into audiological practice. Telepractice is a key feature of this position paper to address issues with regards to communication, education, access to sound, family relationships, attitudes, use of devices, and the underlying consideration of personal factors such as coping strategies and stresses. Organizations offering a range of service delivery models are well placed to meet ICF objectives.

Evaluating Telepractice

This chapter has identified the processes and considerations involved in evaluating telepractice (see Figure 3–1). Identification of stakeholders, evaluation of effectiveness and efficiencies, and identifying implicit aspects of telepractice have been discussed. It is clear there is no single best measure to evaluate telepractice. Attitudes and understanding of stakeholders, cost benefits implications, and technological considerations are all potential barriers (and facilitators) for implementing telepractice. The evidence gathered during implementation of a telepractice service should capture and carefully examine each of these factors and develop strategies to pragmatically address the barriers and find facilitators to address them. Continual review, monitoring, and documentation of the telepractice model implemented through quality assurance programs should continuously introduce facilitators and remove barriers that can provide valuable evidence that telepractice programs can leverage from. It is expected that there is continuous refinement and adjusting of telepractice programs due primarily to changes in technology and an increased experience base.

The first author (Psarros, 2014) has developed a list of barriers and facilitators that have emerged after 3 years of clinical use of telepractice as a model of service delivery (Table 3–5).

Table 3–5. Barriers and Facilitators of Telepractice

Barriers	Facilitators
Organizational attitudes	Positive experiences with clinicians
Consumer choice (recipients, facilitators, local service providers)	Positive experiences with consumers
Reimbursement issues	Cost-effectiveness
Equipment costs	Use of available equipment
Access to remote site to deliver services	Range of sites possible
Privacy and security considerations	Protected Internet access
Stand-alone service	Integration into existing (telepractice) services
Cultural sensitivities	Culturally appropriate
Poor or limited technological literacy	Appropriate health literacy and technical literacy

Although these barriers and facilitators may be tailored for relevance within a particular organizational framework, there is synchrony between what has been reported throughout this chapter and the first author's own clinical experience. Organizational attitudes and consumer choice have been strongly impacted by positive experiences through telepractice, along with increased access to a range of sites. However, currently the lack of reimbursement available presents as a major barrier for the widespread use of telepractice. It is anticipated that the ongoing evaluation of the telepractice model (see Figure 3–1) of service delivery will provide the evidence required for funding to facilitate the sustainability.

Summary

Telepractice requires ongoing evaluation using qualitative and quantitative methods to assess the effectiveness of outcomes and its efficiency, as well as to identify other factors that may emerge through its implementation. Stakeholder characteristics are essential considerations when establishing an evidence base for evaluation of telepractice as a model of service delivery. Evidence must not be limited to recipient outcomes; rather, it should reflect the complex interaction of social, organizational, and human costs and benefits. Sustainable, flexible MOSD must ensure equity of high quality, which could include accessible health care provided through telepractice in isolation or in conjunction with in-person sessions. The dynamic nature of health professions and technology requires a strong collaboration among researchers and practitioners to enable the evidence base for telepractice to be continually built upon. Given the dynamic nature of telepractice, mature programs that have captured the longitudinal evidence base are required to demonstrate the viability of telepractice as a model of service delivery.

References

Abidin, R. R. (1995). *Parenting Stress Index (PSI)* (3rd ed.). Lutz, FL: Psychological Assessment Resources.

Alkmim, M. B., Figueira, R. M., Marcolino, M. A., Cardoso, C. S., Pena de Abreu, M., Cunha, L. R., . . . Antunes, A. P. (2012). Improving patient access to specialized health care: The Telehealth Network of Minas Gerais, Brazil. *Bulletin of the World Health Organisation, 90,* 373–378.

American Speech-Language-Hearing Association. (n.d.). *Telepractice overview.* Retrieved from http://www.asha.org/prpprinttemplate .aspx?folderid=8589934956

Audiology Australia. (2013). *Clinical practice standards.* Retrieved from http://www audiology.asn

Audiology Australia. (2014). *Models of service delivery position paper.* Retrieved from http://www.audiology.asn

Australian Commission on Safety and Quality in Health Care. (2013). *Consumers, the health system and health literacy: Taking action to improve safety and quality* (Consultation paper). Sydney, Australia: Author.

Bakken, S., Grullen-Figueroa, L., Izquierdo, R., Lee, N. J., Morin, P., Palmas, W., . . . Starren, J. (2006). Development, validation and use of English and Spanish versions of the Telemedicine Satisfaction and Usefulness Questionnaire. *Journal of the American Informatics Association, 13,* 660–667.

Bashshur, R. L., & Shannon, G. W. (2009). *History of telemedicine: Evolution, context and transformation.* New Rochelle, NY: Mary Ann Liebert.

Blaiser, K., Edwards, M., Behl, D., & Munoz, K. F. (2012). Telepractice services at Sound Beginnings Utah State University. *The Volta Review, 112,* 365–372.

Botros, A., Banna, R., & Maruthurkkara, S. (2013). The next generation of Nucleus® fitting: A multiplatform approach towards universal cochlear implant management. *International Journal of Audiology, 52*(7), 485–494. doi:10.3109/14992027.2013.781277

Brennan, D. (2013). To move telepractice toward the future, we should look to the past. *Perspectives on Telepractice: Special Interest Group 18, 3*(1), 4–8. Retrieved May 20, 2014, from asha.http.internapcdn .net/asha_vitalstream_com/pubs/.../fullissue.pdf

Brown-Connelly, N. (2002). Patient satisfaction with telemedical access to specialist services in rural California. *Journal of Telemedicine and Telecare, 8,* 7–10.

Cameron, A. M., Bashshur, R. L., Halbritter, K., Johnson, E. M., & Cameron, J. W. (1998). Simulation methodology for estimating financial effects of telemedicine in West Virginia. *Telemedicine Journal, 4,* 125–145.

Clark, M., & Goodwin, N. (2011). *Sustaining innovation in telehealth and telecare* (WSDAN briefing paper). Retrieved from http://bucks

.ac.uk/content/documents/Research/808608/Sustaining-innovation-telehealth-telecare-wsdan-mike-clark-nick-goodwin-october-2010.pdf

Cohn, E. R., & Cason, J. (2012). Telepractice: A wide angled view for persons with hearing loss. *The Volta Review, 112*, 207–226.

Calderon, R., Bargones, J., & Sidman, S. (1998). Characteristics of hearing families and their young deaf and hard of hearing children: Early intervention follow-up. *American Annals of the Deaf, 143*(4), 347–362.

Constantinescu, G., Theodoros, D. G., Russell, T., Ward, E. C., Wilson, S. J., & Wootton, R. (2010). Assessing disordered speech and voice in Parkinson's disease: A telerehabilitation application. *International Journal of Language Communication Disorders, 45*, 630–644.

Dally, K., & Conway, R. (2008). *Invest to grow: Local evaluation report for RIDBC remote early learning program* [Unpublished report]. Callaghan, Australia: University of Newcastle.

Duncan, J. (2008). Telepractice aural habilitation for school aged children. *Perspectives on Aural Rehabilitation and Its Instrumentation, 15*, 1–15.

Eckberg, K., Meyer, C., Scarinci, N., Grenness, C., & Hickson, L. (2012). Family member involvement in audiological appointments with older people with hearing impairment. *International Journal of Audiology.* Advance online publication.

Eikelboom, R. H., Jayakody, D. M. P., Swanepoel, D. W., Chang, S., & Atlas, M. D. (2014). Validation of remote mapping of cochlear implants. *Journal of Telemedicine and Telecare.* Advance online publication. doi:10.1177/1357633X14529234

Griffith, C. (2012, November). Remote servicing helps spread the word to the deaf. *The Australian.* Retrieved from http://www.theaustralian.com.au/business/technology/remote-servicing-helps-the-deaf/story-e6frganx-1226524459829

Hughes, M. L., Goehring, J. L., Baudhuin, J. L., Diaz, G. R., Sanford, T., Harpster, R., & Valente, D. L. (2012). Use of telehealth for research and clinical measures in cochlear implant recipients: A validation study. *Journal of Speech and Hearing Research, 55*, 1112–1127.

Klersy, C., Silvestri, A., Gabutti, G., Raisaro, A., Curti, M., Regoli, F., & Auricchio, A. (2011). Economic impact of remote patient monitoring: An integrated economic model derived from a meta-analysis of randomized controlled trials in heart failure. *European Journal of Heart Failure, 13*, 450–459.

Kopel, H., Nunn, K., & Dosetor, D. (2001). Child and adolescent psychological telemedicine outreach service. *Journal of Telemedicine and Telecare, 7*(Suppl. 2), S235–S240.

Krupinski, E., Norman, C. D., ElNasser, Z., Noyek, A., Ignatieff, A., & Freedman, M. (2011). Successful models for telehealth. *Otolaryngological Clinics of North America, 44*, 1275–1288.

Lewis, C., Packman, A., Onslow, M., Simpson, J., & Jones, M. (2008). A phase II trial of telehealth delivery of the Lidcombe Program of Early Stuttering Intervention. *American Journal of Speech Language Pathology, 17*, 139–149.

Martin, J., & Raine, C. H. (2013). Quality standards in cochlear implants for children and young adults. *Cochlear Implants International, 14*, S13.

May, C., Finch, T., Mair, F., & Mort, M. (2005). Toward a wireless patient: Chronic illness, scarce care and technological innovations in the United Kingdom. *Social Science and Medicine, 61*, 1485–1494.

Mitchell, E. I., Rhodes, L. M., & Grossman, K. (2004, March). Telehealth's promise for the nation's long-term care residents. *Physician Executive*, pp. 52–56.

Morris, M. G., & Venkatesh, V. (2000). Age differences in technology adoption decisions: Implications for a changing workforce. *Personnel Psychology, 53*, 375–403.

Norman, S. (2006). The use of telemedicine in psychiatry. *Journal of Psychiatric and Mental Health Nursing, 13*, 771–777.

Psarros, C. (2014, May). *Home based models of managing implantable technologies: Self-fitting and telepractice.* Paper presented at the XXXII World Congress of Audiology, Brisbane, Australia.

Psarros, C. (2015, April). *The efficiency and effectiveness of telepractice as a model of service delivery in implantable technologies: Meeting the stakeholders needs.* Paper presented at the 10th APSCI conference, Beijing, China.

Psarros, C., van Wanrooy, E., & Pascoe, S. (2012). *Management of cochlear implants using remote technology* (Unpublished internal report). Melbourne, Australia: Hearing Cooperative Research Centre.

Robins, P. M., Smith, S. M., Glutting, J. J., & Bishop, C. T. (2005). A randomized controlled trial of a cognitive-behavioral family intervention for pediatric recurrent abdominal pain. *Journal of Pediatric Psychology, 30*, 397–408.

Rogers, P. (2006). Evidence in action topical paper—Sustainability. *Australian research alliance for children and youth West Perth* cited in Dally, K., & Conway, R. (2008). Invest to grow: Local evaluation report for RIDBC remote early learning program [Unpublished report]. Callaghan, Australia: University of Newcastle.

Ruckdaschel, S., Reiher, M., Rohrbacher, R., & Nagel, E. (2006). The role of health economics in telemedicine. *Disease Management & Health Outcomes, 14*(1), 3–7.

Rushbrooke, E. (2012). Remote mapping for children with cochlear implants (Unpublished master's thesis). Brisbane, Australia: University of Queensland.

Russell, T. (unpublished model). Broad experience and research across 5 domains of telerehabilitation research. Adapted from Fryback, D. G., & Thornbury, R. (1991). The Efficacy of Diagnostic Imaging. *Medical Decision Making, 11*, 88, by Russel at the Telerehabilitation Research Unit, School of Health & Rehabilitation Sciences, The University of Queensland.

Russell, T. G., Buttrum, P., Wootton, R., & Jull, G. A. (2003). Low-bandwidth telerehabilitation for patients who have undergone total knee replacement: Preliminary results. *Journal of Telemedicine and Telecare, 9*(Suppl. 2), 44–47.

Sarant, J., & Garrard, P. (2014). Parenting stress in children with cochlear implants: Relationships among parent stress, child language and unilateral versus bilateral implants. *Journal of Deaf Studies and Education, 19*, 85–106.

Sato, A. F., Clifford, L. M., Silverman, A. H., & Davies, W. H. (2009). Cognitive behavioral interventions via telehealth: Applications to paediatric functional abdominal pain. *Children's Health Care, 38*, 1–22.

Scarinci, N., Worrall, L., & Hickson, L. (2012). Factors associated with third party disability in spouses of older people with hearing impairment. *Ear and Hearing, 33*, 698–708.

Singh, G. (2014). *Teleaudiology: Are patients and practitioners ready for it?* Stäfa, Switzerland: Phonak.

Stith, J., Stredler-Brown, A., Greenway, P., & Kahn, G. (2012). TeleCITE: Telehealth—A cochlear implant therapy exchange. *The Volta Review, 112*(3), 393–402.

Stredler-Brown, A. (2014). Efficacy of telepractice in speech-language pathology. In K. T. Houston (Ed.), *Telepractice in speech-language pathology* (pp. 21–50). San Diego, CA: Plural.

Swanepoel, D. W., & Hall, J. W. (2010). A systematic review of telehealth applications in audiology. *Telemedicine and eHealth, 16*(2), 181–200.

Tang, Z., Weavind, L., Mazabob, J., Thomas, E., Chu-Weininger, M. Y. L., & Johnson, T. R. (2007). Workflow in intensive care unit remote monitoring: A time and motion study. *Critical Care Medicine, 35*(9), 2057–2063.

Theodoros, D. G., Constantinescu, G., Russell, T. G., Ward, E. C., Wilson, S. J., & Wootton, R. (2006). Treating the speech disorder in Parkinson's disease online. *Journal of Telemedicine and Telecare, 12*(Suppl. 3), 88–91.

Victoor, A., Delnoij, D., Friel, D., & Rademaker, J. D. (2012). Determinants of patient choice of healthcare providers: A scoping review. *BMC Health Services Research, 12*, 272.

Waite, M., Cahill, L. M., Theodoros, D. G., Busuttin, S., & Russell, T. G. (2006). A pilot study of online assessment of childhood speech disorders. *Journal of Telemedicine and Telecare, 12*(Suppl. 3), 92–94.

Watzlaf, V. J. M., Fahima, R., Moeini, S., & Firouzan, P. (2010). VOIP for telerehabilitation: A risk analysis for privacy, security and HIPAA compliance. *International Journal of Telerehabilitation, 2,* 1–14.

Wesarg, T., Wasowksi, A., Skarzynski, H., Ramos, A., Gonzalez, J.C.F., Kyriafinis, G., . . . Laszig, R. (2010). Remote fitting in Nucleus cochlear implant recipients. *Acta Oto-Laryngologica, 130*(12), 1379–1388.

Whitten, P., & Love, B. (2005). Patient and provider satisfaction with the use of telemedicine: Overview and rationale for cautious enthusiasm. *Journal of Postgraduate Medicine, 51,* 294–300.

Williams, T., May, C., Mair, F., Mort, M., & Gask, L. (2003). Normative models of health technology assessment and the social production of evidence about telehealth care. *Health Policy, 64,* 39–54.

Wong, L., & Hickson, L. (2012). Evidence-based practice in audiology. In L. Wong & L. Hickson (Eds.), *Evidence-based practice in audiology: Evaluating interventions for children and adults with hearing impairments.* San Diego, CA: Plural.

World Health Organization. (2001). *The international classification of functioning, disability and health (ICF).* Geneva, Switzerland: Author.

World Health Organization. (2010). *Telemedicine: Opportunities and developments in member states: Report on the second global survey on ehealth global observatory for ehealth series.* Retrieved from http://www.who.int/goe/publications/goe_telemedicine_2010.pdf

World Health Organization. (2011). *mHealth (2011): New Horizons for health through mobile technologies.* Retrieved from http://www.who.int/goe/publications/goe_mhealth_web.pdf?ua=1

Wylie, K., McAllister, L., Davidson, B., & Marshall, J. (2013). Changing practice: Implications of the world report on disability for responding to communication disability in under-served populations. *International Journal of Speech-Language Pathology, 15*(1), 1–13.

Young, T. L., & Ireson, C. (2003). Effectiveness of school-based telehealth care in urban and rural elementary schools. *Paediatrics, 112,* 1088–1094.

Zanaboni, P., & Wootton, R. (2012). Adoption of telemedicine: From pilot stage to routine delivery. *BMC Medical Informatics and Decision Making, 12,* 1.

4

Remote Programming of Cochlear Implants

Colleen Psarros and Emma van Wanrooy

Key Points

- Telemapping has the potential to improve equity of access to specialist cochlear implant (CI) services.
- Computer-based CI programming equipment is well suited to telepractice.
- Telemapping has the potential to improve flexibility in models of CI service delivery and has been validated for reliability and feasibility.
- Different technology options are available, and a range of models for delivery of telepractice services has been developed.
- Services can be delivered to cochlear implant recipients of all ages, including those with additional disabilities.
- Future directions in CI services include home-based telepractice and wireless mapping (e.g., remote assistant fitting).

Thirty-five years ago, the landscape of options supporting aural re/habilitation for a person with a severe to profound hearing loss was vastly different than for someone with the same hearing loss today. The collision of technology and hearing loss more than three decades ago with the development of the multichannel cochlear implant (CI) systems has significantly impacted how

91

hearing health practitioners work with individuals with moderate to profound sensorineural hearing loss. Similarly, technology's impact on our daily routines for work, education, and leisure has developed so dramatically that now communication is available in a number of immediate forms in virtually any location. In addition, improvements in cochlear implant technology have supported the extension of candidacy criteria to include people with lesser degrees of hearing loss. This has resulted in an increased number of people who are now eligible to receive a CI. Audiologists are now faced with the challenges of how to serve this growing demographic and the specialized expertise required to ensure successful outcomes. Advancements in information technology and telecommunications provide tools that can be used to address this dilemma. This chapter reviews the rapidly evolving integration of the two frontiers of technology in hearing health care: CIs (and implantable technologies in general) and the use of telepractice. The authors look at how the history of CIs has shaped the current model of service delivery. As well, the authors investigate how hearing health professionals can adapt a model of telepractice to provide efficient and timely services to CI recipients.

Traditional Models of CI Service Delivery

Before considering the integration of telepractice into CI service delivery models, it is critical to understand practices of CI management. Since their commercial development 30 years ago, CIs have become a viable option for providing access to sound for people of all ages with a moderately severe to profound hearing loss (Zeng, Rebscher, Harrison, Sun, & Feng, 2008). A CI is an implantable prosthesis that places electrodes inside the scala tympani of the cochlea that stimulates the auditory nerve through electrical impulses. A signal is sent to the CI through an externally worn speech processor, which has settings unique to each CI recipient. The sound delivered through a CI is determined by the setting of current levels. This setting is achieved by measuring levels of comfortable loudness and, in some devices, additionally through measuring thresholds levels across the electrodes. This is known as the CI "map." The programming of the CI speech processor, sometimes referred to as "mapping," is performed at regular intervals (usually 1, 2, 4, 8, and 12 weeks apart) when the device is first fitted. The map is then reviewed and updated as required every 6 to 12 months for the rest of the recipient's lifetime. Changes in the recipients' "map" may occur due to changes in the biochemical and physiological composition of the cochlea (Newbold, Richardson, Seligman, Cowan, & Shepherd, 2011). Rance and Dowell (1997) note there also can be some postsurgical changes that occur due to the healing mechanisms within the cochlea, such as fibrous sheath growing around the internal electrode array. This sheath can affect the current flow and result in changes in current requirements, which, in some patients, creates the need for regular adjustments of the CI "map" in the acute phase of CI management. Accuracy of mapping may be affected by attention factors and the reliability of responses, particularly in the very young or very old. The settings of a map are verified generally through speech perception testing, questionnaires, or informal observations.

The place of CIs in hearing re/habilitation has grown significantly since their inception. Initially, the candidacy range was quite restricted, and services were provided at only a few locations in a limited number of countries. Patients were often required to travel large distances to obtain services. This is still the case in many areas, as specialist services required for CIs are not available in all countries, and in locations where they are available, access is not always equitable. CI services are generally only available in larger cities (Eikelboom, Jayakody, Swanepoel, Chang, & Atlas, 2014) or via "outreach" services that require the audiologist/hearing professional to travel to different sites. Thus, patients with CIs who do not live close to a major city that has a CI clinic, face numerous access barriers to services for programming and assessment.

Difficulties with travel and the associated cost, possible time away from work or school, and the stress of traveling long distances to CI centers on a regular basis raise many challenges for geographically remote patients and their families. Further, it is not always time- or cost-effective for the professionals providing the "outreach" services to travel to the patients (Krumm, Ribera, & Schmiedge, 2005). In other cases, the barrier may not always be distance. For example, urban patients with social, economic, mobility, or transportation issues also may have difficulty accessing services.

Overall performance with a CI has increased in line with technological improvements and optimization of device fitting, resulting in an expansion in the population for whom a CI is considered a suitable rehabilitation option. Table 4–1 summarizes some of the key advancements in CI research that have influenced the expansion in population of CI recipients.

Along with the expansion in population, advances in technology have influenced changes in the time taken to deliver services related to cochlear implantation. Table 4–2 shows some of the key advancements and potential ways in which services might change in the future given current research being conducted.

CI audiology is continually being influenced by improvements in technology, such as more advanced speech processors and more streamlined methods for measuring maps and creating programs. These changes, in addition to an expanded population of candidates, have led to new ways of assessing and managing clients.

Table 4–1. Features That Have Influenced the Increase in Demand for Cochlear Implants

Feature	Changes Over Time Validated by Research
Technological improvements	Speech coding strategy
	Speech processor technology
	Electrode array design
Electric vs. acoustic vs. combination	Conventional hearing aid compared to cochlear implant
Unilaterally or bilaterally	Bimodal implants
	Bilateral implants
	Electroacoustic devices
Expanded selection criteria	Decrease in age at implantation (infants)
	Increase in age at implantation (elderly)
	Increasing amounts of residual hearing
	Auditory neuropathy spectrum disorder
	Unilateral hearing loss (single-sided deafness)

Table 4–2. Changes That Have Influenced the Delivery of Cochlear Implant Services

	Then (1980s)	Now (2010s)	The Future (2015+)
Preoperative counseling	Limited printed information available Limited base of evidence Very few existing recipients to discuss the process	Online information from manufacturers and other recipients (social media) Printed information available Discussion with professionals and other recipients	Access online—websites, social media More integration of recipients in society 3D modelling of components for counselling
Surgical consultation	Risks and contraindications not completely documented Informed consent based on research data Advised any residual hearing would be lost All consultations face-to-face	Informed consent based on large body of available evidence Focus on hearing preservation Some consultations via video link but majority face-to-face	Continuous evolution of surgical procedures More consultations done by video link
Preoperative assessment	Formal speech perception testing using recorded materials (e.g., MAC battery 4 hours) Promontory stimulation test X-rays and computed tomography scan	Streamlined assessment using more efficient speech perception materials Requiring specialized equipment setup at clinics	Streamlined but standardized assessments performed at a variety of locations with or without telepractice

continues

Table 4–2. *continued*

	Then (1980s)	Now (2010s)	The Future (2015+)
Surgery	6 hours for unilateral Large incision behind ear, hair shaved No preservation of residual hearing	3 hours on average for bilateral cochlear implant (2 hours for unilateral) Small incision behind ear, minimal disturbance to hair Partial/complete preservation of residual hearing in some cases	Preservation of all residual hearing or hair cell regeneration
Mapping	3 hours in total for unilateral map 20 minutes needed to erase the single program 2 hours to do the mapping psychophysics 20 minutes to write the map onto the processor	More advanced mapping software has resulted in more streamlined mapping—approximately 2–10 minutes per ear Automated evaluation of neural telemetry. Psychophysics simplified Progressive programs automatically created Automatic changing of settings to suit acoustic environment	Individualised programming by recipient or their family Link into hearing health care professional for troubleshooting and ongoing monitoring using telepractice or within clinic

	Then (1980s)	Now (2010s)	The Future (2015+)
Equipment for mapping	Desktop computer Floppy disks for patient data Large desktop programming unit	Laptop computer and portable programming unit	Remote control—wireless programming Self-programming
Outcomes measurement and performance monitoring	Live voice, closed-set speech perception assessments	Recorded materials: words and sentences Background noise and speech signal automatically adjusted based on client performance a sound-treated booth Functional evaluations and quality of life questionnaires	Technological advancements allowing speech perception, spatial and qualitative assessments in a wider range of environments more reflective of real world environments
Speech processors	Larger size, body worn, less power efficient Manual controls	Ear level, directional microphones, remote controlled, or automatically adjusted, waterproof or water resistant	Disk shaped (nothing at ear), fully implantable, Bluetooth compatibility

The significant changes in the speech processors, surgical techniques, programming software, and improvements in telecommunications enable telepractice to be a viable option to improve the access of CI services for people living in rural or remote locations and in countries without CI clinics. Paradigms for evaluating CI suitability, surgery, and ongoing management were recently compared across two countries—Germany and the United States—to highlight procedure disparities within the models of CI service delivery (Teschner, Polite, Lenarz, & Lustig, 2012). A number of differences were identified in the components of the multidisciplinary preoperative, perioperative, and postoperative phases of CI service delivery, while the phases of the model for CI management were the same. In age-matched adult populations, they found that there were no significant differences in their speech perception or surgical outcomes. This lends support to the fact that CI models can be described as follows irrespective of the procedures within each phase and the time intervals in which these occur.

Quality standards for cochlear implantation in children and young adults (Martin & Raine, 2013) and for adults (Muller & Raine, 2013) outline the specific phases within the above model (Figure 4–1) with processes adjusted as appropriate for the different populations. Separate quality standards for (re)habilitation of children and adults (Martin, 2013) provide more detail of the ongoing therapy and evaluation over time.

Given that the demand for CI services is expected to continue to increase over coming years with industry growth currently set at 5% (Merrill Lynch, 2014), along with the retention of the existing pool of CI recipients or potential recipients living in locations remote from a CI clinic, alternative models of service delivery need to be investigated, such as telepractice. The World Health Organization (WHO) advocates telepractice as a means of providing access to specialized services as well as delivering education and training of health care providers and the general public (WHO, 2013).

The WHO International Classification of Function (ICF) (WHO, 2001) has set a framework within which a core set of classifications provides a term of reference for describing hearing loss and development of hearing health care. The aim of the WHO ICF is to promote the implementation of activity and participation in audiological practice (Danemark et al., 2009)

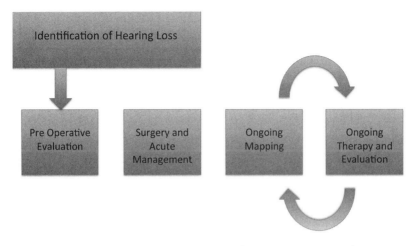

Life Long Management with CI Recipients

Figure 4–1. Phases of a CI model.

(Figure 4–2). This has resulted in a shift from the focus on body function and structure impairment—or hearing loss—to include individuals and families more actively and to generate participation in hearing health care. Access to services is a major consideration of this framework—with telepractice discussed as a viable model of service delivery. Speech-language pathologists (SLPs) have integrated the ICF principles and often advocate more flexibility in the choice of service delivery model used. Telepractice is one of the models of service delivery (Wylie, McAllister, Davidson, & Marshall, 2013). Evidence continues to emerge for the use of telepractice in audiology and is discussed in Chapters 8 and 10 of this book.

Telepractice in CI Service Delivery—Feasibility and Validity

When considering the use of telepractice in CI service delivery, each of the stages of service delivery can be looked at individually. In Figure 4–3 (Psarros, 2015b), the four phases of the CI service delivery model are expanded. The majority of audiological services involved in CI candidacy and management can be

International Classification of Function (ICF)
WHO Hearing Sub Committee (2009)

Body Function	Body Structure	Activity and Participation	Environment
• Hearing Functions • Sound Detection	• Structure of Auditory Nerve • Structure of Cochlea	• Communication • Using Devices • Family Relationships • Education	• Access to Sound • Sound Quality • Attitudes Around Us

Personal Factors: Coping Strategies and Stresses

Figure 4–2. WHO ICF Hearing subcommittee—core sets for hearing loss. Based on Danemark et al. (2009).

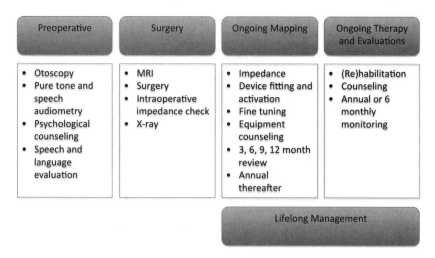

Preoperative	Surgery	Ongoing Mapping	Ongoing Therapy and Evaluations
• Otoscopy • Pure tone and speech audiometry • Psychological counseling • Speech and language evaluation	• MRI • Surgery • Intraoperative impedance check • X-ray	• Impedance • Device fitting and activation • Fine tuning • Equipment counseling • 3, 6, 9, 12 month review • Annual thereafter	• (Re)habilitation • Counseling • Annual or 6 monthly monitoring

Lifelong Management

Figure 4–3. CI model with episodes of service. Based on Psarros (2015a).

delivered remotely from otoscopy to CI programming. Current evidence that validates telepractice for each of these services is discussed.

Telepractice in Preoperative Evaluation

Fabry (2010) reported that the diagnostic application of telepractice in audiology has predominantly focused on otoscopy (used
for visualization and diagnosis of disorders of the ear canal and
eardrum) or on screening for either hearing thresholds or speech
reception thresholds.

Ongoing research by Ter-Horst and Leigh (2012) has investigated the use of telepractice in audiology to conduct air and
bone conduction evaluation of children in rural and remote areas
of Australia. This project used a computer-based audiometer and
videoconferencing using remote access software (all run on a
single laptop computer), a single high-speed Internet connection,
circumaural headphones, and a bone conductor. Protocols were
established that included the development and use of "correction
factors" obtained when children wore occluding headphones.
The results suggested that remote technology and procedures
can assess children's hearing as accurately as conventional face-
to-face assessment. Further, the researchers demonstrated that
sound booths are not necessary to ensure accurate test results,
with careful monitoring of noise levels in the room.

Speech perception testing is an important component of the
management of both pediatric and adult CI recipients (Goehring
et al., 2012). Research into the validity of speech perception
assessments using telepractice is extremely limited at this time.
Speech reception threshold testing using telepractice originated
predominantly with the telephone as the medium for presenting
speech stimuli. This has not included complete diagnostic evaluation of the client. Ribera (2005) successfully administered the
Hearing in Noise Test (HINT) (Nilsson, Soli, & Sullivan, 1994) sentences using telepractice to a group of 20 young adults and found
videoconferencing to be a reliable tool for evaluating speech perception. The researchers reported that there was potential for a
degraded signal with increased Internet activity. Recent attempts
to use videoconferencing for a more comprehensive speech perception evaluation have suggested that future research should
focus on modifications to non-sound-treated environments for
telehealth service delivery in rural areas. A study conducted by
Goehring et al. (2012) showed a negative impact when moving
from a sound-treated room to a quiet office environment. In

addition, this study also compared two sound delivery systems to present the test stimuli but found that neither was sufficiently effective for testing within the remote environment. However, it is likely that the method of stimulus delivery could be modified to improve the signal quality.

Constantinescu (2010) was able to capture good signal quality for patients with Parkinson disease between 54 and 85 years of age to provide speech therapy assessment and speech therapy intervention. This study required highly controlled monitoring of sound pressure level (SPL) and frequency of the speech signal. These factors were critical when evaluating speech perception in individuals with hearing loss, including CI recipients. Results showed that participants who used the remote testing environment were able to achieve similar results on their acoustic and perceptual measures compared to participants who had received their treatment face-to-face. Although some challenges were reported with the remote treatment delivery paradigm, these were compensated for by the clinicians and the participants, and patient satisfaction for the telepractice approach was high.

Telepractice for Intraoperative Monitoring

The application of telepractice for CI management was first documented by Frank, Pengelly, and Zerfoss (2006) with their description of remote mapping and intraoperative monitoring. More recent research has demonstrated the use of remote intraoperative evaluation during CI surgery (Shapiro, Huang, Shaw, Roland, & Lalwan, 2008; Wesarg et al., 2010). Using commercially available software and an intranet (a computer network within an organization) or the Internet, neural response telemetry measures were performed (e.g., measurement of evoked responses from the peripheral part of the auditory nerve stimulated by direct current through individual intracochlear electrodes from the implant array). The authors identified that the main factors that reduced efficiency of this procedure were the slowing of the information transmission through the Internet or that the lesser-trained personnel at the remote location could make errors in setting up the evoked potential equipment. Both of these factors could be overcome, to a degree, through the implementation of training and provision of materials for checking of equipment. Although Internet delays encountered cannot always be accounted for, the use of more robust technology could minimize these issues.

Telepractice in CI Programming— Acute and Long-Term Management

Further reports of the application of telepractice in CI services were provided by Lorens (2009) and Ramos et al. (2009). Ramos et al. (2009) described the use of telepractice with the mapping of adult CI recipients who had been using their devices for 3 months or longer. The researchers reported a greater than 0.5-second delay in the transmission of the stimulus; however, using troubleshooting and emergency stop checks, the researchers ensured that the recipients would not be overstimulated. Lorens (2009) described sessions that were implemented with and without remote mapping and found no significant difference between the two conditions on the parameters assessed. Parents of 114 children and 94 adults and older teenagers with 9 months through 9 years of cochlear implant experience were involved in the study. Questionnaires were presented to recipients and their parents, and they found that there was no reduction in their confidence or rapport with the clinician.

Recent studies conducted under the HEARing Cooperative Research Centre investigating the feasibility of telepractice in CI mapping (Psarros, van Wanrooy, & Pascoe, 2012) demonstrated there were no significant differences between remote mapping of CI recipients of all ages and abilities from one site to another while retaining a high level of user satisfaction (Figure 4–4).

All sessions were conducted with a trained facilitator at the remote site. The initial phase of the study was conducted within the one site for proof of concept before extending to include site-to-site remote mapping. Overall, 70 ears were mapped as part of this feasibility study. As can be seen in Table 4–3, the site-to-site mapping covered distances of up to 4,388 km.

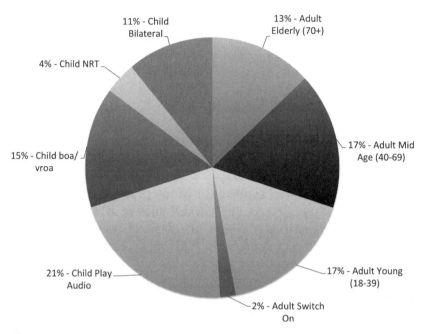

Figure 4–4. Demographics of the 70 ears mapped using telepractice. Based on Psarros et al. (2012).

These findings showed that CI recipients of all ages and abilities could have mapping provided using telepractice with 95% of sessions completed successfully. The 5% that were not completed were due to variability in Internet connection. Time taken for CI mapping was found to be consistent with expected person-to-person intervals within a clinic (e.g., average of 32 minutes for a unilateral map and 40 minutes for a bilateral map) (Figure 4–5). A range of behavioral procedures was used to verify responses of the children and adults, ranging from behavioral observational audiometry (BOA), visual reinforcement audiometry (VRA), conditioned responses or "play audiometry" (Madell & Flexer, 2008), and routine audiometric procedures using a modified Hughson Weslake procedure (Martin, 1986).

A Likert scale questionnaire was administered to the recipient or his or her caregiver, the audiologist, and the facilitator following each section. A rating of 1 = "excellent" and 5 = "poor" was given on a range of experiences that included the picture quality, audio quality, confidence in accuracy of the procedure,

Table 4–3. Site to Site Remote Mapping With the Psarros et al. (2012) Feasibility Study

Mapping Site	Personnel Mapping	Remote Site	Remote Site Personnel	Distance, km	Number of Ears Mapped
Sydney	Audiologist	Port Macquarie	Habilitationist	395	10
Sydney	Audiologist	Newcastle	Audiologist	125	4
Sydney	Audiologist	Darwin	Habilitationist	3,993	6
Sydney	Audiologist	Samoa	Habilitationist/parent	4,388	6
Sydney	Audiologist	Gosford	Habilitationist	90	5
Sydney	Audiologist	Lismore	Audiologist/ habilitationist	725	5
Sydney	Audiologist	Sydney	Habilitationist	15	2

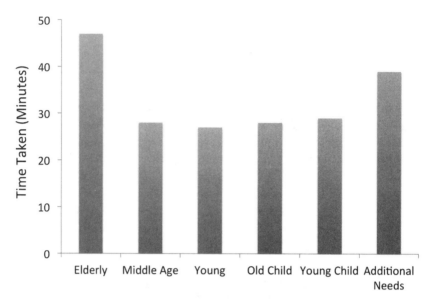

Figure 4–5. Time taken for CI mapping. Based on Psarros et al. (2012).

and overall satisfaction. A rating of 3 or under indicated good satisfaction. As can be seen from Figure 4–6, overall satisfaction for all participants was quite high.

A satisfaction rating between 3 and 1 indicated good satisfaction with the remote mapping procedure; a rating higher than 3 indicated dissatisfaction with the procedure. Overall, CI recipients, audiologists, and the clinicians at the remote site rated their experience with remote mapping as satisfactory. When the recipient group was analyzed further according to age group and ability, ratings for all groups were satisfactory; however, the elderly adults were the least satisfied. This was attributed to their lack of familiarity with the technology, and further investigation of this theory is warranted.

User satisfaction questionnaires are discussed in great detail in Chapter 8. The results need to be considered in light of the health literacy rating of the questionnaires (Bakken et al., 2006). Further, the point at which the survey was administered can impact the outcome, which was observed by Whitten and Love (2005), who observed the possibility of response bias when a survey is administered immediately after the session.

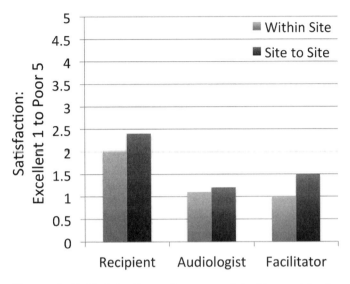

Figure 4–6. Satisfaction ratings completed by recipients, audiologist, and the facilitator of remote CI mapping sessions.

In parallel to this feasibility study, Rushbrooke (2012) conducted a validation study of remote CI mapping with 45 children. Three groups of children were included in the study: 5 for the pilot phase, 20 children aged 5 to 10 years, and another group of 20 children over 10 years of age. Half of the children had remote mapping of their CI in the same building room-to-room and also a face-to-face (FTF) session; the other half had their remote mapping performed over a distance up to 4,000 km as well as an FTF session. Parents of the younger group of children were asked to complete a satisfaction questionnaire.

Rushbrooke (2012) used a specialized computer-based videoconferencing system—the eHAB telerehabilitation system developed at The University of Queensland. This system enables remote consultation between patients and health professionals via a wireless 3G or 4G Internet connection or wide-area network. It uses a virtual private network to provide a secure connection between sites to ensure privacy. A full screen enabled two-way interaction with the client via the eHAB system while the second screen was used to interact with the remote CI programming software (Figure 4–7).

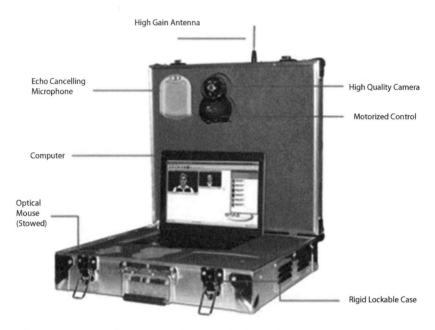

High Gain Antenna

Echo Cancelling Microphone

High Quality Camera

Motorized Control

Computer

Optical Mouse (Stowed)

Rigid Lockable Case

Figure 4–7. eHAB system. NeoRehab Pty Ltd, Brisbane, Australia.

The children's speech perception was assessed using word Consonant Nucleus Consonant words (CNC; Peterson & Lehiste, 1962) or Manchester Junior Words (MJW; Watson, 1957) and Bench-Kowal-Bamford sentences (BKB; Bench & Bamford, 1979). The speech perception testing was performed using both a map created in the remote condition (remote programing) and a map created using the more traditional FTF condition. Speech perception testing results, from these two conditions, were then compared.

Threshold and comfort levels in the recipients CI map were compared to determine if there was a significant difference (i.e., greater than 20% change in the dynamic range). There was a different audiologist performing the mapping in each of the conditions. Paired t tests using group data showed that there was no significant statistical differences for electrode current levels obtained in the maps between FTF and using telepractice. There was no significant difference in speech perception scores for each of the maps. Parent satisfaction questionnaires were generally very positive, with some parents reporting they felt more engaged in the telepractice sessions. Clinicians reported they found the equipment easy to use but reported occasional distortions of the video display. Overall, clinicians felt that the system was advantageous due to benefits of less travel time and the ease of access.

Rushbrooke (2012) found that a fundamental part of the telepractice model was the facilitator. In this study, Rushbrooke noted an appropriate facilitator was someone who could develop good rapport with a child and his or her family, could set up equipment, and could be involved in keeping the child engaged or distracted throughout the mapping task. Most of the studies to date have been limited to specific site-to-site use of telepractice in audiology and have involved a limited range of recipients and personnel. As will be discussed later, further research is required to examine using family members to facilitate telepractice sessions and home-based models of service delivery.

Methodology for Conducting CI Mapping via Telepractice

Telepractice in CI mapping most commonly uses a synchronous model where the client and the audiologist are at separate locations connected via the Internet for communication and for the remote management of the programming software by the audiologist.

As can be seen in Figure 4–8, there is a computer at both sites. The audiologist controls the programming software at the remote site by having remote access to the computer. There is also equipment to enable an audiovisual communication between the two sites. The patient at the remote site is usually accompanied by a facilitator. This can be a trained professional or a caregiver who connects the speech process to the programming hardware. In some cases, the facilitator may be responsible for ensuring clear communication between the audiologist and the client, especially if sound quality between the two sites is poor.

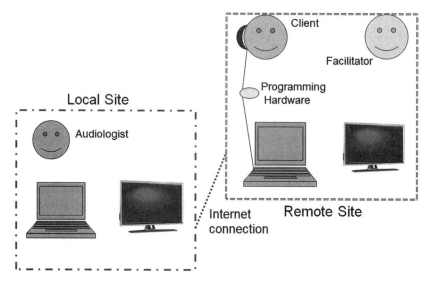

Figure 4–8. Remote CI mapping generic model. Basic remote mapping components. Based on Psarros et al. (2012).

Equipment Requirements for Telepractice

Other than the personnel, there are three essential components required for remote mapping that are in addition to the equipment required for a standard CI mapping appointment. They are as follows:

1. Equipment for an audiovisual link between sites: This can take a number of forms: videoconferencing, readily available free applications such as which may not be appropriate due to privacy regulations or policies, or more specialized programs such as Tandburg MOVI that have the potential to provide a clearer picture by running on a computer network. The vision ideally is displayed separately from the programming software, either on a second monitor or on a tablet device. In addition, there are specialized telemedicine units such as the eHAB.

2. Remote access software between sites: There are multiple applications commonly used in information tech-

nology that can be used for gaining remote access of the computer at the remote site. Some of these are listed in Table 4–4.

3. Internet connection: Minimum requirements are the ability to maintain a stable connection at between 500 and 1,500 kilobits per second upload and download. This can be achieved by a mobile phone with good reception or ADSL lines that are close enough to their local nodes, or most cable or fiber-optic connections. Upload and download capabilities can generally be checked to evaluate the potential impact of distance on the ADSL performance through the Internet provider. An example of this can be found in Table 4–4.

Technology deployed is dependent on the clinic's Internet access and resources. However, availability of Internet access and the communication links may vary within a session. For example, if bandwidth decreases, communication link may move from using video to audio only to preserve the connectivity for

Table 4–4. Essential Components for a Teleaudiology Session

Item	Options
Remote access software to control remote computer	Remote Desktop, Logmein Rescue, Logmein Central, Team Viewer
Video/audio link for communication	eHAB, videoconferencing, telephone, e.g., dedicated VC platform such as Tandburg Movi, & Polycom Real Presence Skype, Microsoft Link, FaceTime
Internet connection	Mobile broadband: 3G or 4G with signal strength greater than –90 dB required OR wired service: ADSL broadband sufficient (365 kBps)
Visual display	Separate monitor from the computer, videoconferencing monitor, tablet (e.g., iPad)/ eHAB

the remote access to the mapping activities. In addition, a fourth component that can facilitate the sharing of client programming files and access to the programming software (instead of loading it onto each computer used at every remote site) is a virtual private network (VPN) or "cloud" technology. This technology provides a safe platform for remote mapping in nonclinical environments as manufacturer software is not loaded onto desktops and cannot be accessed in the clinician's absence. Further, it allows for more streamlining of software updates.

Remote Mapping Procedure

The procedure involved in the remote mapping process can be seen in Table 4–5. It follows the same steps as a standard face-to-face session; however, it is useful for the facilitator to present any live voice speech stimuli or noisemakers that are required to evaluate the map. This prevents distortion to the signal that may occur if stimuli are presented by the audiologist via the video link.

An online training module is available via the HEARnet Learning website that provides frameworks and skills to hearing health care professionals considering the integration of telepractice into remote programming of CIs (Psarros, Rushbrooke, & van Wanrooy, 2013).

This interactive module covers all the fundamentals a hearing health professional would need to implement a telepractice session for CI management, including selection of technology and equipment, resourcing, personnel, and training needs. The module incorporates the technology described in the validation study of Rushbrooke (2012) and the feasibility study of Psarros, van Wanrooy, and Pascoe (2012)). Rushbrooke's use of the eHAB system and Psarros and van Wanrooy's use of "off-the-shelf" equipment that is commonly available in most clinics provide prospective users of telepractice with a variety of options that can be tailored to meet their clinical needs.

Integrated into the training is a reflective exercise to establish an individual's predisposition to using telepractice based on the criteria identified by McCarthy and North (2012). Not all clinicians are adept at using technology in their clinical practice.

Table 4–5. Procedures and Personnel for Cochlear Implant Mapping Using Telepractice

Step	Procedure	Personnel Directly Involved
1	Discuss and review client performance and equipment issues	Remote programmer and programming assistant
2	Impedance check/telemetry measures (neural response telemetry/auditory response telemetry/neural response integrity optional)	Remote programmer
3	Threshold measurement (where indicated)	Remote programmer (and programming assistant as required)
4	Loudness level setting	Remote programmer
5	Live mode check	Remote programmer (and programming assistant as required)
6	Map verification through speech (e.g., six sounds, words, sentences)	Remote programmer and programming assistant
7	Repeat if bilateral mapping	As above
8	Write information to sound processors	Remote programmer
9	Explain session outcome	Remote programmer (and programming assistant if required)
10	Session write-up	Remote programmer

Source: Based on Psarros, Rushbrooke, and van Wanrooy (2013).

Reflecting on factors that could impact service delivery provides insights into potential barriers to successful implementation. Tips and hints on how to manage clients of different age groups and abilities, as well as troubleshooting of technology, have been captured in the guidelines and online training module. A comprehensive troubleshooting guide is available online to accompany the training module and printable guidelines for remote mapping. Most manufacturers of CIs have provided information on their websites regarding telepractice. To date, there are limited printed resources available providing detailed guidelines for CI mapping except for manufacturer specific recommendations.

Future Directions in Remote Programming of CIs

Wireless Modules for CI Programming

With recent advances in CI programming, basic mapping is possible via a remote control with some speech processors, rather than via programming hardware. Adult recipients, older children, and caregivers of younger children can use the Nucleus CR110 to perform auto neural response telemetry(NRT) to evaluate the threshold for the neural response, adjust the comfort levels with the master volume, and adjust bass and treble to generate a map (Botros, Banna, & Marruthurakka, 2013). This is using the remote assistant fitting (RAF) procedure. When applying this technology in a telepractice model, rather than having specialized programming equipment, mapping is done via the remote assistant.

As can be seen in Figure 4–9, using the RAF method removes the need to access a computer at the remote end, but a video link is still required. Video cameras are in place so that the audiologist has a clear view of the display on the remote to guide the appropriate setting of maps. The audiologist instructs the facilitator at the remote site which buttons to press on the remote assistant. Limitations to this method include the following:

- Reduction in access to the speech spectrum through excessive reduction of bass and/or treble by the client after a mapping session
- Inability to measure individual T and C levels by the audiologist to fine tune the map
- Possible uncomfortable sound percepts during the administration of the NRT

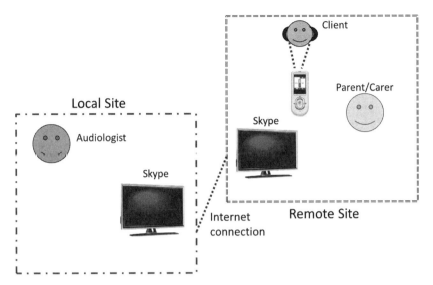

Figure 4–9. Telepractice using the RAF procedure. Remote RAF components. Based on Abrahams, Neal, and Lavery (2014).

Thus, it is most likely that the RAF procedure would be used to supplement other service delivery options, such as face-to-face maps or a remote CI map where the client is connected to the programming software.

Telepractice in the Home

Ongoing management of CI recipients requires (re)habilitation to maximize the integration of the auditory signal into communication contexts. Children require regular intervention to facilitate the development of speech and language. Home-based interventions provide the natural environment specific to the child and family's needs (Sato, Clifford, Silverman, & Hobart-Davies, 2009). The use of telepractice to provide habilitation for children with hearing loss has been well documented in the literature (Constantinescu et al., 2014; Houston & Stredler Brown, 2012). Guiding principles for telepractice with children who have vision or hearing loss have been developed for this purpose (McCarthy & North, 2012). This home-based model of service delivery has excellent application for consideration when extending telepractice to CI mapping.

Hughes et al. (2012) found that the personnel required to facilitate the remote mapping session (at the client site) potentially may only be needed to set up the equipment, which ordinarily could be the client themselves or a significant other. Using a family-centered model, inclusion of parents into a remote mapping session in the role of facilitator is a possibility. Rushbrooke (2012) observed that "with the correct selection criteria and training a non-clinician could assist at the recipient end and this has the potential to increases the scope for this technology significantly" (p. 65). In keeping with Rushbrooke's observations, the Royal Institute for Deaf and Blind Children (RIDBC) has implemented a home-based telepractice CI program. The RIDBC teleschool has been in operation for 10 years. Over that time, more than 800 families from around Australia and internationally have benefited from telepractice services delivered to their home. The majority of families have access to contemporary videoconferencing equipment, with some families using Skype or FaceTime.

Home-based CI management began at RIDBC in 2013, and data are being collected on the efficacy of this procedure. Data collected include the patient and clinician satisfaction, completion of mapping sessions, monitoring of speech perception outcomes, ongoing speech and language evaluations, functional listening questionnaires, data logging for Nucleus 6 recipients, and review of impedance and mapping levels. The majority of sessions are performed in collaboration with the RIDBC teleschool consultant, who is at the local end with the audiologist, while the child and family are at the remote site. The role of the consultant is to provide behavioral reinforcement where appropriate (e.g., visual reinforcements such as puppets or digital images). Children were aged 7 months to 6 years when implanted through this program. There are 10 families who have been implanted through the RIDBC program utilizing the home-based telepractice model. Of these, three alternate with FTF sessions, hence blending the service they are accessing. A number of families who live in regional and remote areas have transferred to the RIDBC program in order to access the home-based service. Data collection also occurs with these children. It is the intention of this project to gather data and develop a mature program that carefully evaluates the longitudinal effects of a telepractice method of CI programming. Initial findings have shown variability in the Internet connection between different geographical locations. However, recipient satisfaction has been quite high (Figure 4–10).

Comments from participants have been overwhelmingly positive. The main negative comments were regarding the occasional issues with use of the Internet. In those situations, the resolution of the videoconferencing is decreased to preserve the bandwidth for the CI mapping.

Logistics regarding shipping of cables and equipment to families requires careful planning. Families report this is preferable to having to organize to travel—in some cases, this would involve plane travel to cover the 3,900 km from the CI center. The CI programming software is installed and accessed using cloud technology discussed earlier in this chapter. The next step in this

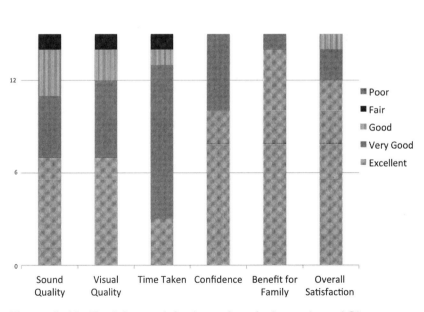

Figure 4–10. Recipient satisfaction ratings for home-based CI programming using telepractice at RIDBC. Based on Psarros, van Wanrooy, and Pascoe (2012).

process is to investigate methods of evaluating the CI program. A study is under way to investigate the use of functional questionnaires and speech perception evaluations for this purpose.

Eikelboom et al. (2014) have developed a PC-based system that can be used for remote mapping of CIs and speech perception testing that could be readily implemented in the home environment with the recipient potentially facilitating the session. There is great value in investigating the feasibility of a home-based model, particularly for families living in areas where a clinic for CI mapping is not easily accessible or in countries where this service is not available at all.

Blending Face-to-Face Sessions With Telepractice

"One size does not fit all," hence the importance of considering a blended model of CI service delivery where telepractice and person-to-person sessions complement each other (Figure 4–11). Ideally, this is tailored to the recipient and his or her family's needs.

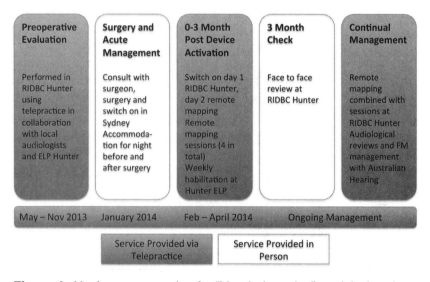

Figure 4–11. A case example of a "blended service" model whereby a child has a mix of telepractice management for audiological and educational service as well as within-clinic person-to-person services. Based on Psarros (2015b).

Summary

CI services have expanded dramatically over the past 30 years, and the demand for services is expected to continue to increase. Telepractice provides the means to increase the availability of CI services to those people who do not have easy access to a specialized clinic. In addition, it opens up the possibility of implementing more flexible models of service delivery that cater to the needs of clients and their families. In the future, greater adoption of tools such as the RAF procedure is expected as well as an increase of home-based and blended models of service delivery for both mapping and (re)habilitation.

References

Abrahams, Y., Neal, K., & Lavery, S. (2014, May). *Wireless, portable, paediatric cochlear implant fitting via the Nucleus Remote Assistant: Transforming service delivery.* Paper presented at XXXII World Congress of Audiology, Brisbane, Australia.

Bakken, S., Grullen-Figueroa, L., Izquierdo, R., Lee, N. J., Morin, P., Palmas, W., . . . Starren, J. (2006). Development, validation and use of English and Spanish versions of the Telemedicine Satisfaction and Usefulness Questionnaire. *Journal of the American Informatics Association, 13*, 660–667.

Bench, J., & Bamford, J. M. (1979). *Speech hearing tests and the spoken language of hearing impaired children.* London, UK: Academic Press.

Botros, A., Banna, R., & Marruthurakka, S. (2013). The next generation of Nucleus Fitting: A multiplatform approach towards universal cochlear implant management. *International Journal of Audiology, 52*, 485–494.

Constantinescu, G. (2010). *Disordered speech and voice in Parkinson's disease using a PC based telerehabilitation system* (Unpublished doctoral thesis). Brisbane, Australia: University of Queensland.

Constantinescu, G., Waite, M., Dornan, D., Rushbrooke, E., Brown, J., McGovern, J., . . . Hill, A. (2014). A pilot study of telepractice delivery for teaching listening and spoken language to children with hearing loss. *Journal of Telemedicine and Telecare, 20*, 135–140.

Danemark, B., Kramer, S., Hickson, L., Gange, J. P., Moeller, C., Swanepoel, D. W., & McPherson, B. (2009). *Development of ICF core sets for hearing loss.* Oldenberg, Germany: International Collegium of Rehabilitative Audiology.

Eikelboom, R. H., Jayakody, D. M. P., Swanepoel, D. W., Chang, S., & Atlas, M. D. (2014). Validation of remote mapping of cochlear implants. *Journal of Telemedicine and Telecare.* Advance online publication. doi:10.1177/1357633X14529234

Fabry, D. (2010, September/October) Applications of telehealth for hearing care. *Audiology Today,* pp. 18–25.

Frank, K., Pengelly, M., & Zerfoss, S. (2006). Telemedicine offers remote cochlear implant programming. *Voices, 13,* 16–19.

Goehring, J., Hughes, M., & Baudhin, J. (2012). Evaluating the feasibility of using remote technology for cochlear implants. *The Volta Review, 112*(3), 255–265.

Goehring, J., Hughes, M., Baudhuin, J., Valente, D., McCreery, R. W., Diaz, G. R., . . . Harpster, R. (2012). The effect of technology and testing environment on speech perception using telehealth with cochlear implant recipients. *Journal of Speech and Hearing Research.* Advance online publication. doi:10.1044/1092-4388(2012/11-0255

Houston, K. T., & Stredler Brown, A. (2012). A model of early intervention for children with hearing loss provided through telepractice. *The Volta Review, 112,* 283–296.

Hughes, M. L., Goehring, J. L., Baudhuin, J. L., Diaz, G. R., Sanford, T., Harpster, R., & Valente, D. L. (2012). Use of telehealth for research and clinical measures in cochlear implant recipients: A validation study. *Journal of Speech and Hearing Research, 55,* 1112–1127.

Krumm, M., Ribera, J., & Schmiedge, J. (2005). Using a telehealth medium for objective hearing testing: Implications for supporting rural universal newborn hearing screening programs. *Seminars in Hearing, 26,* 3–12.

Lorens, F. (2009, May). Telemedicine: Cost benefit for patients, e-learning for doctors. *Congress Tribune Issue, 3,* 4.

Madell, J., & Flexer, C. (2008). *Paediatric audiology: Diagnosis, technology and management.* New York, NY: Thieme Medical.

Martin, F. (1986). *Introduction to audiology* (3rd ed.). Englewood Cliffs, NJ: Prentice-Hall.

Martin, J. (2013). Quality standards for (re)habilitation. *Cochlear Implants International, 14*(Suppl. 2), S34–S38.

Martin, J., & Raine, C. H. (2013). Quality standards for cochlear implantation in children and young adults. *Cochlear Implants International, 14*(Suppl. 2), S13–S20.

McCarthy, M., & North, J. (2012). *RIDBC Teleschool: Guiding principles for telepractice.* Sydney, Australia: North Rocks Press.

Merrill Lynch. (2014). *Equity Australia Medical Specialty report.* Sydney, Australia: Cochlear Ltd.

Muller, J., & Raine, C. H. (2013). Quality standards for adult cochlear implantation. *Cochlear Implants International, 14*(Suppl. 2), S6–S12.

Newbold, C., Richardson, R., Seligman, P., Cowan, R., & Shepherd, R. (2011). Electrode stimulation causes rapid changes in electrode impedance of cell-covered electrodes. *Journal of Neural Engineering, 8,* 3.

Nilsson, M., Soli, S. D., & Sullivan, J. (1994). Development of the hearing in noise test for the measurement of speech reception thresholds in quiet and in noise. *Journal of the Acoustical Society of America, 95,* 1085–1099.

Peterson, G. E., & Lehiste, I. (1962). Revised CNC lists for auditory tests. *Journal of Speech and Hearing Disorders, 27,* 62–70.

Psarros, C. (2014). *CI model with episodes of service* [Unpublished report]. Melbourne, Australia: Hearing Cooperative Research Centre Project.

Psarros, C. (2015a, April). *New models of service delivery at SCIC.* Paper presented at 10th APSCI conference, Beijing, China.

Psarros, C. (2015b, April). *The efficiency and effectiveness of telepractice as a model of service delivery in implantable technologies: Meeting the stakeholders needs.* Paper presented at the 10th APSCI conference, Beijing, China.

Psarros, C., Rushbrooke, E., & van Wanrooy, E. (2013). *Remote cochlear implant mapping. HEARnet on-line learning module.* Melbourne, Australia: Hearing Cooperative Research Centre.

Psarros, C., van Wanrooy, E., & Pascoe, S. (2012). *Management of cochlear implants using remote technology* [Unpublished report]. Melbourne, Australia: Hearing Cooperative Research Centre Project.

Ramos, A., Rodrigues, C., Martines-Beneyto, P., Perez, D., Gault, A., Falcon, J., & Boyle, P. (2009). Use of telemedicine in the remote programming of cochlear implants. *Acta Otolarnygologica, 129,* 533–540.

Rance, G., & Dowell, R. C. (1997). Speech processor programming. In G. M. Clark, R. S. C. Cowan, & R. C. Dowell (Eds.), *Cochlear implantation for infants and children: Advances* (pp. 147–170). San Diego, CA: Singular.

Ribera, J. (2005). Interjudge reliability and validation of telehealth applications in a hearing in noise test. *Seminars in Hearing, 26,* 13–18.

Rushbrooke, E. (2012). *Remote MAPping for children with cochlear implants* (Unpublished master's thesis). Brisbane, Australia: The University of Queensland.

Sato, A. F., Clifford, L. M., Silverman, A. H., & Hobart-Davies, W. (2009). Cognitive behavioural interventions via telehealth: Applications to paediatric functional abdominal pain. *Children's Health Care, 38,* 1–22.

Shapiro, W., Huang, T., Shaw, T., Roland, T., & Lalwan, A. (2008). Remote intraoperative monitoring during cochlear implant surgery is feasible and efficient. *Otology and Neurology, 4,* 495–498.

Ter-Horst, K., & Leigh, G. (2012, April). *Remote assessment of hearing: Paediatric hearing assessment using tele-audiology—An investigation in rural and remote populations.* Paper presented at the Hearing CRC Annual Review, Melbourne, Australia.

Teschner, M., Polite, C., Lenarz, T., & Lustig, L. (2012). Cochlear implants in different health care systems: Disparities between Germany and the US. *Otology and Neurootology, 34,* 66–72.

Watson, T. J. (1957). Speech audiometry for children. In A. W. G. Ewing (Ed.), *Educational guidance and the deaf child* (pp. 278–296). Manchester, UK: The University Press.

Wesarg, T., Wasowksi, A., Skarzynski, H., Ramos, A., Gonzalez, J. C. F., Kyriafinis, G., . . . Laszig, R. (2010). Remote fitting in Nucleus cochlear implant recipients. *Acta Otolaryngologica, 130,* 1379–1388.

Whitten, P., & Love, B. (2005). Patient and provider satisfaction with the use of telemedicine: Overview and rationale for cautious enthusiasm. *Journal of Postgraduate Medicine, 51,* 294–300.

World Health Organization. (2001). *International classification of functioning, disability and health.* Geneva, Switzerland: Author.

World Health Organization. (2013). *Multi country assessment of national capacity to provide hearing care.* WHO ICF Hearing Sub-Committee. Retrieved from http://www.icf-research-branch.org/download/finish/11-other-health-conditions/171-brief-icf-core-set-for-hearing-loss

Wylie, K., McAllister, L., Davidson, B., & Marshall, J. (2013). Changing practice: Implications of the World Report on Disability for responding to communication disability in under-served populations. *International Journal of Speech-Language Pathology, 15,* 1–13.

Zeng, F. G., Rebscher, S., Harrison, W. V., Sun, X., & Feng, H. (2008). Cochlear implants: System design, integration and evaluation. *IEEE Review of Biomedical Engineering, 1,* 115–142.

5

Remote Diagnostic Hearing Assessment

Robert H. Eikelboom and De Wet Swanepoel

Key Points

- Diagnostic teleaudiology is a key component of a broader teleaudiology service.
- Synchronous, asynchronous, or mixture of these models can be employed for a teleaudiology service.
- Equipment for diagnostic teleaudiology has been shown to be reliable and accurate.
- Well-supported local support staff are required as facilitators for teleaudiology.

One of the emerging challenges in global health is the high prevalence of hearing loss across all ages and the acute shortage of hearing health professionals to diagnosis and manage hearing loss. Furthermore, the location of populations in greatest need for services and the location of trained hearing health professionals are mismatched. Following a similar pattern is the prevalence of ear disease and the access to specialist ear health services. The increasing life expectancy globally also can be expected to place more demands on hearing health services, as the number of people with age-related hearing loss increases.

Telehealth technologies have been promoted as a mode of bridging the distance between the unserved and hearing health specialists. Aided by the exponential growth in communication networks, especially in developing countries, many hearing health assessment services can now be effectively delivered by telehealth. However, many aspects do need to be put in place to deliver effective services, from referral processes to human resources to the choice of equipment.

An important element in ear and hearing health is the aspect of diagnostic audiometry. For the purposes of this chapter, diagnostic audiometry includes all aspects related to the assessment of hearing thresholds, including a clinical history, otoscopy, tympanometry, air and bone conduction audiometry with masking, speech perception audiometry, and discussions with the patient. Neonatal screening or assessment, pediatric play audiometry, screening audiometry, and intraoperative monitoring are not considered.

What Is the Need?

The World Health Organization (WHO, 2013) estimated that the global population with disabling hearing loss is almost 360 million people and that 32 million of these are children. Disabling hearing loss for adults is defined at a mean hearing threshold of 40 dB or greater in the better hearing ear; for children, the threshold is 30 dB or greater. The highest prevalence (over 6.1% of the population) is found in central and subcontinental Asia and some eastern European countries. At the second tier of prevalence (between 4.4% and 6.1%) are Central America, the Caribbean islands, South America, sub-Saharan Africa, and most of Southeast Asia.

Access to hearing health professionals is generally inversely associated with the prevalence of disabling hearing loss in a population (Fagan & Jacobs, 2009; Goulios & Patuzzi, 2008). Many countries with the greatest prevalence have little or no documented access to ear health care professionals. This pattern can also be reflected on a national level, where those living in rural and remote areas face a greater disease burden and poorer access to clinical services, as the distribution of audiologists and otolaryngologists per person and per square kilometer reduces significantly as remoteness increases (Table 5–1).

Table 5–1. ENTs and Audiologists in Australia by Remoteness Index

	ENTs		Audiologists	
	/100,000 Population	/1,000 km²	/100,000 Population	/1,000 km²
Major cities	24.1	25.3	57.4	60.33
Inner regional	14.5	0.29	33.6	0.67
Outer regional	0	0	15.3	0.04
Remote	0	0	30.6	0.01
Very remote	0	0	0	0

Source: Adapted from Australian Bureau of Statistics 2006 Census and Australian Institute of Health and Welfare 2009 Medical Labour Workforce data.

Overview of Teleaudiology Model(s) for the Delivery of Diagnostic Hearing Assessment

Two modes of telehealth service delivery models and a combination of the two can be utilized in delivery of diagnostic hearing assessments. The synchronous model, also known as the live model, provides a real-time connection between the parties to a telehealth consultation. Computer and communication equipment enables the clinician to remotely control some of the equipment used for diagnostic assessment. Videoconference facilities enable voice and video communication between the patient and the clinician. Live telehealth is often used for counseling patients when no objective assessments take place and also for education and professional development when patients are not involved.

Synchronous teleaudiology provides the most personal mode of consultation besides a face-to-face consultation. Clinicians can interact directly with a patient and his or her family, provide immediate advice, and include the attending clinician in the consultation. Live telehealth does require good communication infrastructure that includes a network capacity (bandwidth) that can provide good-quality video and voice signals. Quality of service (QoS) is a descriptor that is used at times to describe the reliability and quality of the communication channel. There are some limitations. In most cases, infrastructure does not have the capacity to provide live high-resolution images from, for example, a video-otoscope. This requires a high QoS where bandwidth is high and is guaranteed. Furthermore, live telehealth requires efficient scheduling for all parties to the consultation to be present; this is not always possible in health systems, especially when health services are delivered opportunistically rather than being planned.

The asynchronous model for telehealth, also known as store-and-forward, refers to services that do not involve the simultaneous presence of all parties who are normally in a clinical consultation. Clinical information is gathered and stored, then sent for review to a clinician, who in turn will normally send information back to the originating clinic. The clinical information collected may include hearing screening results, diagnostic audiograms, a clinical history, video-otoscope images, newborn hearing results, or middle ear assessment (tympanometry, Otoacoustic Emissions [OAEs]). It is suited to a number of situations, typically when the communications infrastructure does not support live telehealth, when clinical appointments are difficult to schedule or the timing is unpredictable, or when the collection of data is time-consuming and can easily be performed by trained health workers.

There is a case to be made for utilizing a mixed model, incorporating both synchronous and asynchronous modes of teleaudiology. Typically, this would involve a local health worker conducting tests and collecting data in an asynchronous mode and for live telehealth to be utilized for counseling or to remotely conduct audiological testing (Biagio, Swanepoel, Adeyemo, Hall, & Vinck, 2013; Lancaster, Krumm, Ribera, & Klich, 2008).

Does Assessment by Telehealth Provide the Same Outcomes as Face-to-Face Assessment?

Validation studies are essential in order to provide confidence that a telehealth service does not provide inferior outcomes. Although variability is inherent in behavioral testing, including in air and bone conduction audiometry, there is an expectation that the variability between telehealth-based audiometry and remote audiometry is not greater than the reliability and variability of traditional modes of audiometry. International standards (ISO 8253-1) indicate that the uncertainty in thresholds is at least ±5 dB for frequencies 4 kHz and less and even greater for higher frequencies.

The validity of aspects of remote diagnostic air and bone conduction audiometry has been reported in a number of studies (Choi, Lee, Park, Oh, & Park, 2007; Eikelboom, Swanepoel, Motakef, & Upson, 2013; Givens et al., 2003; Krumm, 2007; Margolis, Glasberg, Creeke, & Moore, 2010; Swanepoel & Biagio, 2011; Swanepoel, Koekemoer, & Clark, 2010). The first group relates to comparing manual audiometry conducted in either the conventional face-to-face mode or manual audiometry conducted by synchronous telehealth. The early work was conducted by Givens and colleagues (2003), who showed variations of thresholds of between 0.0 and 1.3 dB across the 250- to 8,000-Hz test frequencies. When examining the percentage of thresholds of participants in a study with variations of less than 5 dB, Choi and colleagues (2007) reported 89% in 31 subjects; Swanepoel et al. (2010) reported 96% in 30 subjects, most of whom had normal hearing; and Krumm (2007) reported 97% in 30 normal-hearing subjects.

The second group arises from the recent interest in automated audiometry as a way to facilitate asynchronous telepractice models. Automated audiometry adopts the standard procedures to determine air and bone conduction thresholds (Eikelboom et al., 2013; Margolis et al., 2010; Swanepoel & Biagio, 2011). However, being automated in nature, it potentially releases the need for this testing to be undertaken by an audiologist, allowing instead for a trained health worker to administer the test. It has therefore been advocated for teleaudiology (Swanepoel, Olusanya, & Mars, 2009). A comprehensive review of automated audiometry (Mahomed, Swanepoel, Eikelboom, & Soer, 2013) has shown that the difference between manual and automated audiometry is comparable to the test-retest variability of both manual audiometry and automated audiometry.

One of the challenges of conducting air and bone conduction audiometry outside of audiology clinics is the control of the ambient sound level. At least two automated audiometry systems have addressed this by using sound-occluding headsets. The AMTAS utilizes the Sennheiser HDA 200 headset and has performed well in a validation study that included people with a hearing loss tested in a quiet room rather than a sound-treated booth (Eikelboom et al., 2013). The KUDUwave (Figure 5–1) uses a custom-built over-the-ear headset, plus insert earphones (Swanepoel et al., 2010). In addition, the device monitors the environmental sound and can pause testing if the levels are too high. Like the AMTAS, the KUDUwave has been shown to be suitable to be used in quiet rooms.

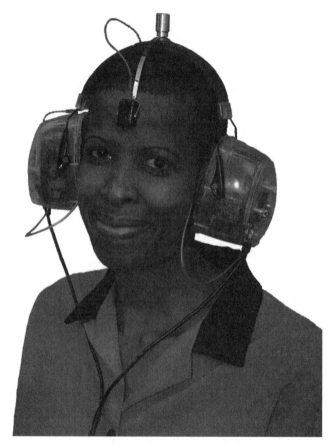

Figure 5–1. KUDUwave custom-built over-the-ear headset, plus insert earphone.

Recommendations for Successful Outcomes

Technology Requirements

Synchronous and asynchronous telehealth have different technology requirements. The synchronous mode requires a moderately fast and reliable network connection for an audiologist to remotely control equipment.

A fast and reliable network connection is required to achieve high-quality voice and video communication. Commonly available tools such as Skype (Microsoft, Redmond, Washington, USA), Teamviewer (TeamViewer GmbH, Göppingen, Germany), and Hangouts (Google Inc.) can provide this facility. However, even high-speed network connections may suffer from delays in transmission and dyssynchrony between voice and video. Although this may at best be annoying to normal-hearing people, they are likely to cause significant problems for those with hearing loss. Live video-otoscopy similarly will require a very high-speed network connection and has to date only been achieved with dedicated communication channels. Firewalls are often put in place by institutions as a security measure. Gaining entry into the organization's network will usually require some high-level negotiations.

Audiological Equipment Requirements

The choice of audiometer depends on the telehealth model adopted. For live telehealth implementations, an audiometer that can be controlled by a computer must be selected. Models from various manufacturers are available. Remote control is normally achieved by "remote desktop" software; PC-Anywhere (Symantec Corporation, Mountain View, California, USA), Teamviewer (TeamViewer GmbH, Göppingen, Germany), and Remote Desktop Services, also known as Terminal Services (Microsoft, Redmond, Washington, USA), have all been used for this purpose. They all display the computer screen on the computer screen of the remote clinician and allow the clinician to use his or her computer mouse and keyboard. Some attention is required to set this up, including providing permission for control of a computer to be ceded to another user. A limitation may be that data are saved on the computer at the site of the audiometer and printouts of the results are not normally available to the clinician; making this available to the clinician requires some additional steps.

For store-and-forward implementations, an automated audiometer is required. The choice is presently limited. Although a number of devices have been validated, only one is commercially available (KUDUwave, Eyemoyodotnet, South Africa). Some manufacturers include an automated option with the software for their audiometer (e.g., MedRX, Largo, Florida, USA), but information on validation is not available.

The otoscope and tympanometry are also important tools for a diagnostic telehealth. The choice of a standard otoscope is straightforward but should be selected to provide a good clear view and have replaceable speculums.

A video-otoscope is a very useful tool for telehealth. Live images may be shared by others—patient, family members, other clinicians—in the room and with a suitable network connection also to another site. Images can be stored for later review and asynchronous transmission to another site.

The choice of video-otoscope is more complex as there are instruments available across a wide price range and of varying quality (Mbao, Eikelboom, Atlas, & Gallop, 2003). Furthermore, their choice should be governed with safety in mind; rod telescope-based video-otoscopes are unsuitable as they can be potentially unsafe in unskilled hands. In general terms, better images are obtained with more expensive instruments. Judgements should be made on quality of image (encompassing focus, field of view, color, and resolution of image), ease of use, connectivity to a computer, and software provided. A fixed-focus instrument may be preferable to one that requires manual focusing as the latter is difficult, if not potentially unsafe, when this is performed with the device in the ear.

The choice of tympanometry should be made on the basis of ease of use, including reporting of results, and access to service and calibration services. Some devices are able to capture data directly into a computer, but this may not be useful if not integrated into the rest of the telehealth software. Others provide a printout that can provide a permanent record of results. These can be scanned to provide an electronic record.

Speech perception testing via telehealth is currently problematic in a synchronous telehealth model of delivery. This is due to the degradation of the quality of voice signals when videoconferencing and the challenges in setting up a calibrated testing environment at the patient site. In an asynchronous model, if the correct testing environment can be provided, a trained assistant co-located with the patient will be able to administer a speech perception test. Automated speech perception tests have been successfully used as part of a hearing screening program (Smits, Merkus, & Houtgast, 2006). However, diagnostic speech audiometry has as yet not progressed much beyond a research phase and will have to rely on forced-choice answers (Kapteyn, 1969; Stevenson, 1975) or reliable speech recognition software to recognize responses by patients.

Other Nontechnical Requirements

The local assistant is key in most aspects of teleaudiology. This assistant is required to set up the equipment, including placing equipment (e.g., headphones on the patient) and assist with the instructions. The assistant will also use some of the equipment that the remote audiologist is not able to control, for example, the otoscope and tympanometer.

Otoscopy will be required to identify possible contraindications to tympanometry and audiometry. The assistant will have to be trained to recognize these contraindications, such as obstructions in the ear canal, external ear disease, discharge, or tympanic membrane perforation. Video-otoscopy images can be captured and sent to the remote clinician for assessment (Biagio et al., 2013; Eikelboom, Mbao, Coates, Atlas, & Gallop, 2005). Tympanometry results can be transposed onto a form or a printout incorporated into the patient record.

The skill of this person will vary; for example, a local general audiologist may be assisting in the consultation with a remotely located specialized hearing implant audiologist, or a health worker or nurse may assist with switching on an audiometer and fitting a headset on a patient for a remotely based audiologist to perform audiometry.

A clinical history is an important element in a telehealth consultation. In the case of live telehealth, this can be performed by the clinician. However, in asynchronous telehealth settings, it is preferable to utilize a pro-forma developed in consultation with the clinical team. In situations where the prevalence of ear disease is high, the clinical history may include questions related to discharge, pain, dizziness, and associated risk factors (e.g., head injury, prematurity).

A comprehensive protocol should also be developed by the whole team. This should define the referral pathway; the use of all equipment, including calibration and maintenance requirements; testing protocols; the responsibility of all members in the telehealth; and training requirements. In some jurisdictions, general telehealth protocols may already be in place that should be used.

Environmental Challenges

A number of environmental challenges may present themselves. Assessment of hearing thresholds strictly requires certified sound-treated environments to control ambient noise levels. In situations where this is not possible, the following solutions are suggestions:

- Measurement of the average environmental noise levels and taking this into account when determining the minimum expected hearing levels that can reliably be recorded
- Use of circumaural headphones or insert earphones for greater attenuation of ambient noise
- Choosing as quiet a place as possible, and testing in quiet periods during the day, or pausing until temporary noise levels pass
- Using an automated audiometer that has been validated (i.e., AMTAS or KUDUwave) and operated in either manual or automated mode

Telehealth is often associated with remote areas that may pose extreme environmental conditions such as heat or cold, humidity, and dust, as well as rough road conditions when traveling to sites. Sensitive equipment should be packed in protective cases and used only within the specified operating conditions.

Humidity-controlling materials (e.g., desiccant such as silica gels) can be used to absorb moisture when equipment is packed away.

Training Requirements

Training is essential for all participants in diagnostic teleaudiology service. This should encompass the use of all the equipment, including the communication tools. In addition to initial training, regular support should also be included in the program. In some cases, participants may be coming from a low threshold (e.g., health workers with no previous experience in hearing health). For these, all the new information can easily be overwhelming. Initial training sessions should ideally be accompanied by a few days of close supervision in a clinical setting as well as support calls or visits short periods afterward.

The referral pathway and operational protocols should also be familiar to all those involved. For those new to ear and hearing health, providing some background information on the cause, nature, and effects of hearing loss and ear disease can be valuable for them to gain an appreciation of the value of their work. Some basic diagnostic skills also will be valuable. For example, if a moderate to severe hearing loss is determined, they will be able to modify the way they communicate verbally with the patient. If otoscopy and/or tympanometry reveals a perforation, they can ensure that the perforation is properly captured in a video-otoscope image.

Follow-Up Care

The referral process is a vital element in diagnostic teleaudiology. The operational protocols should clearly state who is responsible for the patient in any telehealth consultation. It is normally advised that the patient remains the responsibility of the clinic and clinicians at the physical site of the patient, with the remote clinician acting as a consultant (Wade, Eliott, & Hiller, 2012).

The consulting clinicians can, however, provide comprehensive advice if they are confident that the results are a valid representation of a face-to-face consultation. Should some doubt exist, then they can request that tests be repeated, and if possible, tests can be consulted live.

The consulting clinician currently has a number of options for follow-up care. Counseling of patients can be provided via a live videoconference session. These can be used to discuss the management options. If hearing aids are indicated, it may be possible for behind-the-ear hearing aids to be provided. However, to date there is little supporting documentation that these can be fitted remotely. One company website (http://www.ototronix diagnostics.com/intellifit) does offer a remote fitting service, but no published validation information is available. Although this is a current limitation with diagnostic teleaudiology, there is much value in providing this service. For those where rehabilitation with a device is not indicated, unnecessary travel can be avoided, and the patient can be provided with more timely advice. Where intervention is indicated, arrangements can be made for the most suitable mode of delivery.

In cases where ear disease is present, the consultant audiologist will be able to refer the patient to a local general practitioner. The results from diagnostic teleaudiology may also be useful for local speech pathology services.

Tips and Hints

A number of challenges should be considered when planning and implementing teleaudiology services.

QoS is used to describe the performance of an Internet connection and includes issues such as delays, bandwidth, and availability. In most situations, the QoS is such that it may affect live telehealth consultations (Hughes, Hudgins, & MacDougall, 2004). This will result in breakup or delays in voice and video communication and degradation of signal quality.

Privacy and security of data should be maintained, and most jurisdictions will have protocols to assist designing teleaudiology systems. Key considerations are as follows:

■ Management of data, which includes defining which data should be retained and in what form

- Sharing of data, defining how data are transferred between organizations and individuals
- Security of data and systems, ensuring that only those authorized are allowed access to data

Most jurisdictions will have guidelines and protocols regarding privacy and security of data. HIPPA (Health Insurance Portability and Accountability Act) is the most prominent of these.

Although the technology required to deliver most teleaudiology services is available, and validity has been demonstrated, a system will only be as good as the people who are involved in delivering the service. "Buy-in" from local clinicians and support staff is essential but also from the clinicians who are involved in the assessment, diagnosis, and management of patients. Similarly, the perceptions of audiologists and patients about telehealth may need to be shifted. However, evidence suggests that patients are more willing to utilize telehealth services (Eikelboom & Atlas, 2005; Eikelboom, Jayakody, Swanepoel, Chang, & Atlas, 2014) than clinicians (Wade, Eliott, & Hiller, 2014).

Potential for This Model of Service Delivery

The service outlined here does have the potential to improve the access to services to people with hearing loss. At this stage, technology for diagnostic audiometry means that only calibrated equipment can be used, and therefore services will still have to be delivered to designated sites, such as hospital clinics, public health clinics, and allied health sites (e.g., pharmacies). An assistant is still required for almost all aspects of diagnostic audiology (i.e., tympanometry and otoscopy). In the future, the assessment of thresholds may be further simplified and automated such that individuals may perform the test by themselves. Further in the future, diagnostic and imaging techniques may also reduce the need for current middle ear assessment techniques and manual otoscopy. Already home-based otoscopy has been advocated (https://cellscope.com/). Clinical histories may be taken in computer-assisted diagnostic systems (Goggin, Eikelboom, & Atlas, 2007).

What Are the Barriers to Increased Uptake From Hearing Health Professionals?

Although there is sufficient evidence to show that the technology solutions exist, and that there is a need for the provision of diagnostic audiology by telehealth, there are few reports of its efficacy. Services focused on ear disease have been shown to be effective as a model, to reduce waiting times, and to reduce costs. No such studies have been reported for audiology services.

A number of factors probably at play are currently restricting uptake:

- Workload: With the current worldwide undersupply of audiologists, there is little incentive for audiologists to consider an additional form of service delivery that will generate even more work.
- Human factors: Automated audiometry may have a strong role in teleaudiology. However, despite now having a relatively long history of providing proven equivalent assessment of thresholds as manual audiometry, there has been little uptake of automated audiometry in clinical practice. It has the potential to save costs and allow audiologists to focus on more valuable use of their time. Education about the validity of teleaudiology practices will be required.
- Awareness: The introduction of telehealth services is often patient driven or driven by local health workers (Doarn et al., 2008). Patients will therefore have to be aware of the option of teleaudiology services in order to raise a demand. Education of the population and health workers in underserviced areas is therefore important for services to be initiated and developed.
- Support: Associated with awareness is also support for the introduction of teleaudiology services from health service organizations. Particularly in underserviced areas, there are usually competing demands from many other areas of health. This indicates a role for national and international professional bodies such as the Interna-

tional Society of Audiologists and the World Health Organization in promoting the urgency of hearing health.

■ Gaps in service delivery models: As already indicated, there are few options for the local delivery of hearing rehabilitation. This may be a current disincentive for developing teleaudiology services.

Summary

Teleaudiology has the potential to provide access to ear and hearing health services to many people who current face barriers to services and also change the way that clinicians do their work. Diagnostic teleaudiology is an important element of a broader teleaudiology service, which may include pediatric and adult screening, counseling, and management. Most of the technological requirements for diagnostic teleaudiology have been shown to be reliable and accurate, and the key role of local support staff has been demonstrated. The form of the teleaudiology service, whether it is a synchronous, asynchronous, or a mixed model, can be designed to meet the local requirements. Further research is required to explore the barriers to the uptake of diagnostic teleaudiology.

References

Biagio, L., Swanepoel, D., Adeyemo, A., Hall, J. W., III, & Vinck, B. (2013). Asynchronous video-otoscopy with a telehealth facilitator. *Telemedicine Journal and e-Health*, *19*, 252–258.

Choi, J. M., Lee, H. B., Park, C. S., Oh, S. H., & Park, K. S. (2007). PC-based tele-audiometry. *Telemedicine Journal and e-Health*, *13*, 501–508.

Doarn, C. R., Yellowlees, P., Jeffries, D. A., Lordan, D., Davis, S., Hammack, G., . . . Kvedar, M. D. (2008). Societal drivers in the applications of telehealth. *Telemedicine Journal and e-Health*, *14*, 998–1002.

Eikelboom, R. H., & Atlas, M. D. (2005). Attitude to telemedicine, and willingness to use it, in audiology patients. *Journal of Telemedicine and Telecare*, 11(Suppl. 2), S22–S25.

Eikelboom, R. H., Jayakody, D. M. K., Swanepoel, D., Chang, S., & Atlas, M. D. (2014). Validation of remote mapping of cochlear implants. *Journal of Telemedicine and Telecare, 20*, 171–177.

Eikelboom, R. H., Mbao, M. N., Coates, H. L., Atlas, M. D., & Gallop, M. A. (2005). Validation of tele-otology to diagnose ear disease in children. *International Journal of Pediatric Otorhinolaryngology, 69*, 739–744.

Eikelboom, R. H., Swanepoel, D., Motakef, S., & Upson, G. S. (2013). Clinical validation of the AMTAS automated audiometer. *International Journal of Audiology, 52*, 342–349.

Fagan, J. J., & Jacobs, M. (2009). Survey of ENT services in Africa: Need for a comprehensive intervention. *Global Health Action, 2.* doi:10.3402/gha.v2i0.1932

Givens, G. D., Blanarovich, A., Murphy, T., Simmons, S., Blach, D. & Elangovan, S. (2003). Internet-based tele-audiometry system for the assessment of hearing: A pilot study. *Telemedicine Journal and e-Health, 9*, 375–378.

Goggin, L. S., Eikelboom, R. H., & Atlas, M. D. (2007). Clinical decision support systems and computer-aided diagnosis in otology. *Otolaryngology-Head and Neck Surgery, 136*, S21–S26.

Goulios, H., & Patuzzi, R. B. (2008). Audiology education and practice from an international perspective. *International Journal of Audiology, 47*, 647–664.

Hughes, G., Hudgins, B., & MacDougall, J. (2004). Using telehealth technology to improve the delivery of health services to people who are deaf. *Conference Proceedings of the IEEE Engineering in Medicine and Biology Society, 4*, 3084–3087.

Kapteyn, T. S. (1969). A four choice pictorial test in relation to speech-audiometry. *International Journal of Audiology, 8*, 652–653.

Krumm, M. (2007). Audiology telemedicine. *Journal of Telemedicine and Telecare, 13*, 224–229.

Lancaster, P., Krumm, M., Ribera, J., & Klich, R. (2008). Remote hearing screenings via telehealth in a rural elementary school. *American Journal of Audiology, 17*, 114–122.

Mahomed, F., Swanepoel, D., Eikelboom, R. H., & Soer, M. (2013). Validity of automated threshold audiometry: A systematic review and meta-analysis. *Ear and Hearing, 34*, 745–752.

Margolis, R. H., Glasberg, B. R., Creeke, S., & Moore, B. C. (2010). AMTAS: Automated method for testing auditory sensitivity: Validation studies. *International Journal of Audiology, 49*, 185–194.

Mbao, M. N., Eikelboom, R. H., Atlas, M. D., & Gallop, M. A. (2003). Evaluation of video-otoscopes suitable for tele-otology. *Telemedicine Journal and e-Health, 9*, 325–330.

Smits, C., Merkus, P., & Houtgast, T. (2006). How we do it: The Dutch functional hearing-screening tests by telephone and Internet. *Clinical Otolaryngology, 31*, 436–440.

Stevenson, P. W. (1975). Responses to speech audiometry and phonemic discrimination patterns in the elderly. *Audiology, 14*, 185–231.

Swanepoel, D., & Biagio, L. (2011). Validity of diagnostic computer-based air and forehead bone conduction audiometry. *Journal of Occupational and Environmental Hygiene, 8*, 210–214.

Swanepoel, D., Koekemoer, D., & Clark, J. (2010). Intercontinental hearing assessment: A study in tele-audiology. *Journal of Telemedicine and Telecare, 16*, 248–252.

Swanepoel, D., Mngemane, S., Molemong, S., Mkwanazi, H., & Tutshini, S. (2010). Hearing assessment-reliability, accuracy, and efficiency of automated audiometry. *Telemedicine Journal and e-Health, 16*, 557–563.

Swanepoel, D., Olusanya, B. O., & Mars, M. (2009). Hearing health-care delivery in sub-Saharan Africa—A role for tele-audiology. *Journal of Telemedicine and Telecare, 16*, 53–56.

Wade, V. A., Eliott, J. A., & Hiller, J. E. (2012). A qualitative study of ethical, medico-legal and clinical governance matters in Australian telehealth services. *Journal of Telemedicine and Telecare, 18*, 109–114.

Wade, V. A., Eliott, J. A., & Hiller, J. E. (2014). Clinician acceptance is the key factor for sustainable telehealth services. *Qualitative Health Research, 24*, 682–694.

World Health Organization. (2013). *Millions of people in the world have hearing loss that can be treated or prevented.* Geneva, Switzerland: Author.

6

Remote Hearing Aid Fittings

David A. Fabry

Key Points

- Approximately 80% of potential hearing aid candidates do not have access to hearing health care professionals.
- Remote hearing aid fittings are a viable alternative approach.
- Remote hearing aid fittings have the potential to improve access, efficiency of service delivery, and market penetration.
- Digital hearing aid technology enables remote programing.
- Increased prevalence of hearing loss, low market penetration, and changing demographics provide considerable opportunities for remote hearing aid fittings around the world.

Remote hearing aid fittings provide an alternative approach to the traditional hearing aid distribution process that may be used to increase hearing aid market penetration in both developed and developing countries by providing improved access to hearing health care professionals, improved efficiency for service and delivery of hearing aids, and lower costs for private and public distribution. This chapter discusses the current and future global hearing aid markets within this context.

Global Population Estimates of Hearing Loss

According to World Health Organization (WHO) estimates from 42 population-based studies (WHO, 2012), there are 360 million persons worldwide (5.3% of the world's population) with "disabling" hearing loss who would benefit from the use of amplification. Disabling hearing loss refers to hearing loss greater than 40 dB in the better hearing ear in adults (15 years or older) and greater than 30 dB in the better hearing ear in children (0–14 years). As many as 80% of all those with disabling hearing loss live in areas where they have little or no access to hearing health professionals (Swanepoel et al., 2010). Furthermore, hearing loss is a "cradle to grave" issue: 328 million (91%) of those with hearing loss are adults (183 million males, 145 million females), and 32 million (9%) are children. Approximately one third of persons over 65 years of age are affected by disabling hearing loss; most are in South Asia, Asia Pacific, or sub-Saharan Africa.

The Global Hearing Aid Market

Currently, approximately 11 million hearing aids are sold per year worldwide; the vast majority are digital or digitally programmable devices. The six largest hearing aid manufacturers collectively hold a total market share of 90%; the main markets are Organisation for Economic Co-operation and Development (OECD) nations. As Figure 6–1 illustrates, 41% of all devices are dispensed in Europe, followed by 29% in North America, 21% in the Asian Pacific, 7% in South America, and 2% in Africa. Figure 6–2 illustrates hearing aid market penetration rates globally; Australia, the United States, and the European Union have the highest percentage of those with measureable hearing loss using amplification, but none exceed 40%.

Geographic market unit split

Majority of hearing aids sold in developed markets

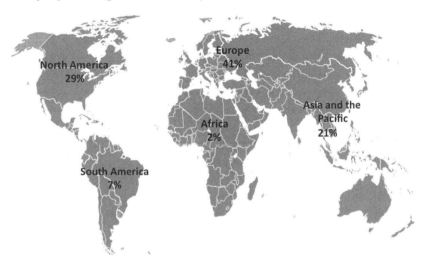

Figure 6–1. Percentage of hearing aids dispensed as a function of total units.

Penetration rates

Percentage of hearing-impaired population wearing hearing aids

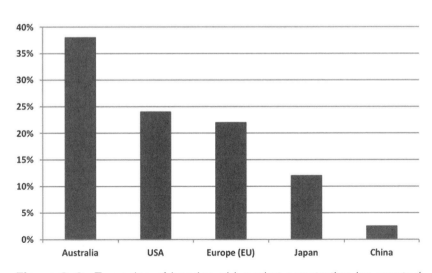

Figure 6–2. Examples of hearing aid market penetration by country/ region.

Hearing Aid Users in Transition

The average age of first-time hearing aid users is approximately 70 years. Binaural hearing aid fitting rates vary dramatically by country; for example, nearly 80% in the United Kingdom are fit with two hearing aids, while 70% in Japan are fit monaurally. Globally, the market is transitioning from pre–World War II era patients to the "baby boom" generation born between 1946 and 1964. In the United States, baby boomers comprise 80 million (25% of the U.S. population) and account for 75% to 80% of U.S. wealth. Boomers constitute 35% to 38% of Internet users; with 42% of today's seniors (over 65 years) online, this percentage is set to increase even more.

Growth Opportunity

The combination of increased prevalence of hearing loss, low market penetration, and changing demographics provides considerable opportunity for the hearing aid market globally. In addition, the fact that nearly all hearing aids sold today are digital means that they interface, either by "wired" or "wireless" connection, to some form of programming device, which offers the possibility of "remote" programming of hearing aids. This provides advantages for improving service and delivery in both developed and developing nations by providing access for hard-of-hearing patients to hearing health care professionals.

West et al. (2010) reported on the opportunity to improve efficiency within the Veterans Administration by reducing travel times for veterans who live in urban, rural, or highly rural environments by setting the following goals:

- Primary care: 70% of urban or rural veterans should have to travel no more than 30 minutes if they are urban or rural residents or more than 1 hour if they are highly rural.
- Acute care: 65% should travel no more than 1 hour if they are urban, 90 minutes if rural, and 2 hours if highly rural.

■ Tertiary care: 65% should travel no more than 2 hours if they are urban or rural residents or beyond Veterans Integrated Service Network (VISN) boundaries if they are highly rural.

Based on data collected regarding actual travel times experienced by veterans, which greatly exceeded these goals, it appears as though there is significant opportunity to improve services for rural and highly rural veterans via telehealth for hearing aid follow-up and/or fitting.

Applicable Modes of Telehealth for Remote Hearing Aid Fitting

Both synchronous and asynchronous modes of service provision may be employed with remote hearing aid programming, although "real-time" synchronous models will most likely be employed for initial fitting and adjustment, with "cloud-based" approaches being used for postfitting adjustments. Real-time methods provide clinicians and patients with greater opportunity for interaction and engagement during the fitting process that parallels the "face-to-face" environment currently in place. The barrier to remote fitting is resistance to change the "status quo" by both clinician and patient due to perceived technology limitations. Properly managed, remote hearing aid fitting and follow-up care provide the potential for a modern-day "Pangaea" to remove barriers and distance to the roughly 80% of potential hearing aid candidates that do not have access to hearing health care professionals. There are, nonetheless, obstacles to achieving success with telehealth and hearing aid fitting.

Barriers to Success With Remote Hearing Aid Fitting

Reimbursement

Today, not all telehealth costs are reimbursed in the United States, which is problematic for some, but not all, aspects of audiology diagnostic and rehabilitative services. This is less of a consequence for hearing aid fitting, given that in most cases, these services are not covered by third-party reimbursement and are often "bundled" into the cost of the hearing aid.

In general, however, reimbursement for telehealth services is a challenge globally. Medicare, which has set the standard for the U.S. health care market, reimburses for telehealth services when the "originating" site (where the patient is at the time of service) is in rural or medically underserved areas, defined by the U.S. Department of Health and Human Services as a "Health Professional Shortage Area" (http://datawarehouse.hrsa.gov/) or county that is outside of any Metropolitan Statistical Area (MSA), defined by the Health Resources and Services Administration and the Census Bureau, respectively. The originating site must be a "medical facility" and not the patient's home. "Medical facilities" include private practices, offices, hospitals, and rural health clinics. This reimbursement is not affected by the "remote" site (the location of the practitioner). Currently, Medicare only pays for real-time interactive telehealth services that mimic normal face-to-face interactions between patients and their health care providers. Medicare does cover cloud-based asynchronous applications, such as teleradiology and remote EKG applications, as they do not typically involve direct interactions with patients. Medicare does cover asynchronous telehealth applications in Alaska and Hawaii, presumably due to their being more geographically remote from the contiguous 48 states.

There is currently no single widely accepted standard for private insurance payers. A few insurance companies recognize the potential for telehealth and will reimburse a wide variety of services. The majority of insurers, however, have yet to develop comprehensive reimbursement policies, and so payment for telehealth may require approval prior to treatment in order to be reimbursed. Similarly, reimbursement for telehealth services via Medicaid services varies across states, so clinicians are advised to check with the major insurance companies and the Medicaid program in their state to get a definitive answer and policy regarding coverage for real-time and cloud-based telehealth services.

Licensing and Credentialing Issues

Another barrier for telepractice programs and remote hearing aid fitting relates to licensure. Many states require health care providers to be licensed to practice in the originating site's state. Therefore, with limited exceptions, telehealth consultations with an audiologist across state lines require licensing paperwork and/or exceptions to be made. One approach, in response to nursing shortages across the United States, has been the development of the Nurse Licensure Compact (NLC). The process for creating the NLC began in 1996 to remove regulatory barriers and increase access to safe nursing care by establishing an interstate compact that supersedes state laws in participating states (currently 23 states recognize the NLC). This mutual recognition model allows a nurse to have a single license (in his or her state of legal residence) and to practice in other states (both physical and electronic) subject to each state's practice law and regulation. The latter part of this requirement distinguishes the NLC from national certifications that have been used in the past to define audiologist proficiency by placing the responsibility for ensuring minimum patient care requirements at the state license board level rather than a national professional organization. Although not perfect, it serves as one example of a model agenda for audiology telehealth service. Another, the Federation of State Medical Boards (FSMB), is a nonprofit organization comprising 70 medical licensing and disciplinary boards that acts as a collective voice for continuous improvement of health care standards for physician practice (http://www.fsmb.org/). In 2000, the FSMB established the Special Committee on License Portability, ultimately resulting in the development of A Model Act to Regulate the Practice of Medicine Across State Lines, which developed a specific policy to address state reciprocity for medical licensure, including provisions that require annual registration with the state license board to permit interstate practice of medicine within the state (e.g., https://www.revisor.mn .gov/statutes/?id=147.032). Although a significant departure from current physician licensure, it still places ultimate responsibility on state licensure boards to ensure that quality of patient outcome is not compromised for its residents. Another related issue concerns the accreditation of hospitals and clinics providing patient privileges for health care practitioners who are involved with primary or follow-up care via telemedicine. The U.S. Centers for Medicare & Medicaid Services (CMS) proposed new regulations in May 2010 that would permit accredited hospitals to accept the credentialing and privileging of practitioners offering telehealth services from another accredited facility (credentialing "by proxy"), rather than requiring each hospital to independently credential and privilege each provider. The flexibility provided under this new proposed rule would minimize the duplicative nature of the process for hospitals that provide telehealth services to Medicare patients. Although not specific to audiology, this proposed ruling telegraphs the intentions of CMS to streamline and modernize the provision of Medicare and Medicaid services to patients via telemedicine. A copy of the proposed rule is available at http://www.americantelemed.org/files/public/policy/Fed_Reg_C_P%281%29.pdf. In summary, the issues related to licensure and accreditation are dynamic and evolving rapidly; practitioners are advised to check with their state license board and accreditation specialist prior to offering telehealth services across hospitals and state lines.

Guidelines for Clinician-Patient Interactions

The American Telemedicine Association (ATA) published core operational guidelines for telehealth services involving provider-patient interactions in 2014 (http://www.americantelemed.org/resources/standards/ata-standards-guidelines/core-operational-guidelines-for-telehealth-services-involving-provider-patient-interactions#.U43Xk15X9g1). These guidelines provide an update to the previously published *Core Standards for Telemedicine Operations* (November 2007) and cover fundamental requirements to be followed when providing health care services using telecommunications technologies and other electronic communications among patients, practitioners, and other health care providers.

Remote Hearing Aid Fitting Examples

Fabry (1996) demonstrated clinical utility for hearing aid adjustments to patients in remote locations. More recently, Ferrari and Bernardez-Braga (2009) made remote probe-tube measurements (using a technician) on 60 patients aged 18 to 84 years and demonstrated test-retest reliability within 3 dB for frequencies between 250 and 6000 Hz. The feasibility and accuracy of remote hearing aid fitting are proven; the essential ingredient is to determine the best way to implement a practical model for use with hearing patients.

Implementation of Remote Hearing Aid Fitting

Location Requirements

As defined above, the "originating" site, where the patient is located at the time of service, must currently be a "medical" facility to be considered for Medicare reimbursement. If this is not a consideration, then the originating site may be a clinic, nursing home, residence, or any other location that meets the physical and telecommunication requirements listed below. The "remote" location, where the clinician is located, could also be a medical facility, private practice or retail location, or possibly a residence as well but should provide a "professional" appearance.

Telecommunication Needs

For synchronous telehealth applications, real-time communication requirements have included T1, broadband, or DSL access at both locations, if audio and video communication is desired. More recently, the possibility has been introduced for use of mobile phones, which now outnumber humans on the planet. In the United States, 96% of the population owns a mobile phone, of which 56% are smartphones. Furthermore, 43% of adults aged 65 years or older, with incomes in excess of $75,000, own a smartphone (http://www.pewinternet.org/Reports/2013/Smart phone-Ownership-2013/Findings.aspx). Mobile phone applications are likely the most promising platform for widespread use of telehealth as it relates to hearing aids.

For asynchronous applications, any telecommunication carrier that can handle data communication will suffice, although slower transmission rates will impact clinical efficiencies.

Computing Needs

Both the originating and remote locations must have access to hardware (e.g., computer, tablet, mobile phones) that may be used to connect to the Internet and communicate with other devices. In addition, both locations must have access to software that may be used to connect to the Internet and communicate with other devices (e.g., computers, tablets, cell phones). Also, the originating location must have access to software that allows authorized access by the remote location to "control" software and hardware applications necessary for "wired" or "wireless" programming of hearing aid features.

Hearing Aid Programming Needs

In 2014, 80% of all hearing aids dispensed in the United States allowed wireless programming, which minimizes hardware applications at the originating location, but some hardware, cabling, and expertise are still necessary. Typically, the "hardware" for hearing aid programming is most commonly accomplished via the following methods:

- Hi-PRO Box: a dedicated interface that couples to a computer via RS-232 serial port or USB connector
- NOAH-LiNK: a wireless programmer that connects to a computer via USB port or dedicated wired/wireless programmer

More recently, wireless hearing aids have been introduced that use Bluetooth Low Energy (BLE) or Bluetooth 4.0 to communicate directly between the device and a mobile phone. This promising approach has already led to the development of "Made for iPhone" and "Made for Android" platforms. No technical expertise is required beyond the ability to "pair" the device to a mobile phone. In turn, this would allow a professional to take control of the device remotely, with the user's permission, to employ a traditional "professional-driven" synchronous fitting or follow-up session where the clinician and patient are connected via Skype, FaceTime, Gotomeeting or other teleconferencing programs.

Clinician-Driven Versus Patient-Driven
Hearing Aid Fitting Approaches

One of the most intriguing possibilities for the role of telehealth in the hearing aid fitting process relates not to the initial fit but the optimization of fitting parameters to "real-world" listening environments. Presently, this is one of the more challenging situations encountered by both the clinician and patient, as the clinical environment is often a poor substitute for everyday situations. Certainly, clinicians may attempt to simulate background noise, reverberation, and increased talker-listener distance in the clinical setting, but unless they are willing to make "house calls," patients may find it a poor substitute for the real thing.

Now, smartphones may be used to enable patients to assist with the fine-tuning of initial hearing aid settings by adjusting bass, treble, and other hearing aid characteristics in the actual environment where they have difficulty. Some applications even allow the patient to "geo-tag" those settings to a specific location via the smartphone's internal GPS coordinate system. This feature uses a combination of synchronous (patient-adjusted response) and asynchronous (clinician-monitored response) that represents an ideal hybrid approach to provide high impact, lowers clinical costs, and may be executed rapidly, which are hallmarks of the "Blue Ocean" business strategy (Kim & Mauborgne, 2005) to create an uncontested market space. At present, telehealth is underutilized in the audiology (and health care) community, but it provides a tremendous opportunity for patient engagement and clinical efficiency.

Summary

Remote hearing aid fitting has been well documented in the literature as a viable alternative to "face-to-face" programming for initial hearing aid fitting and follow-up. Very few technical barriers remain regarding this technology; perhaps the biggest hurdles are faced by the clinician's ability to give up "control" of the hearing aid fitting process by allowing remote-fit, patient-driven fittings and fine-tuning to challenge the role of the practitioner.

The oldest "baby boom" generation patients are just reaching the average age of first-time hearing aid users. Much has been written about the emergence of the boomers and the impact on the hearing aid market, but one thing is true: whenever they become the dominant force of any consumer or health care segment, they change the market to meet *their* needs. Telehealth provides an opportunity for clinicians to provide convenient, efficient access for hearing aid fitting, and the biggest barrier appears to be the status quo. The time is now.

References

American Telemedicine Association. (2014). *Core operational guidelines for telehealth services involving provider-patient interactions.* Retrieved from http://www.americantelemed.org/resources/standards/ata-standards-guidelines/core-operational-guidelines-for-telehealth-services-involving-provider-patient-interactions#.U43Xk15X9g1

Fabry, D. A. (1996, November). *Remote hearing aid fitting applications.* Paper presented at the 8th Annual Mayo Clinic Audiology Videoconference Rochester, MN.

Ferrari, D. V., & Bernardez-Braga, G. R. (2009). Remote probe microphone measurement to verify hearing aid performance. *Journal of Telemedicine and Telecare, 15*(3), 122–124.

Kim, W. C., & Mauborgne, R. (2005). *Blue ocean strategy: How to create uncontested market space and make the competition irrelevant.* Cambridge, MA: Harvard Business School Press.

Swanepoel, D. W., Clark, J. L., Koekemoer, D., Hall, J. W., Krumm, M., Ferrar, D. V., . . . Barajas, J. J. (2010). Telehealth in audiology: The need and potential to reach underserved communities. *International Journal of Audiology 49*(3), 195–202.

U.S. Department of Health and Human Services. (2014). *Health professional shortage area.* Retrieved from http://datawarehouse.hrsa.gov/

West, A. N., Lee, R. E., Shambaugh-Miller, M. D., Bair, B. D., Mueller, K. J., Lilly, R. S., . . . Hawthorne, K. (2010). Defining "rural" for veterans' health care planning. *The Journal of Rural Health, 26*(4), 301–309.

World Health Organization. (2012). *WHO global estimates on prevalence of hearing loss: Mortality and burden of diseases and prevention of blindness and deafness.* Geneva, Switzerland: Author.

7

Telerehabilitation in Audiology

Michelle von Muralt, Lynda Farwell, and K. Todd Houston

Key Points

- Intervention and rehabilitation after fitting of hearing technology is essential to achieving the best communication outcomes for individuals with hearing loss.
- Services delivered through distance communication (e.g., telepractice, teleintervention, telerehabilitation) allow greater equity of access and a more flexible range of service options for children and adults with hearing loss.
- Telerehabilitation offers solutions to the barriers that children and adults with hearing loss experience when seeking out services with qualified professionals.
- Initial research into the satisfaction and outcomes achieved using a telepractice model of rehabilitation indicates that it is a viable and equitable service compared to face-to-face (i.e., in-person) intervention options.

The fitting of hearing technology is only the first step in facilitating a successful intervention process for children and adults with hearing loss. Habilitation or rehabilitation after fitting of hearing aids or implantable technologies (e.g., bone conduction implants, middle ear implants, and cochlear implants) is essential to maximize functional outcomes for each patient (Boothroyd,

2007; Moeller, 2010; Tye-Murray, 2009; Yoshinaga-Itano, Sedey, Coutler, & Mehl, 1998). To achieve optimal listening and spoken language outcomes after hearing technology is fitted, it is important that a patient engages with an experienced, trusted, and qualified habilitation professional to maximize his or her listening skills and communication (Estabrooks, Houston, & McIver-Lux, 2014; Gagne, 2000; Tye-Murray, 2009). This intervention should be provided by professionals with specific knowledge of, and training in (re)habilitation services for individuals with hearing loss (Houston, 2014a; Joint Committee on Infant Hearing [JCIH], 2007). Speech-language pathologists, teachers of the deaf, and audiologists are all able to offer habilitation services to children. Adults with hearing loss typically receive rehabilitation services from qualified speech-language pathologists and audiologists. Families of young children with hearing loss who have chosen a listening and spoken language approach, such as auditory-verbal therapy, may struggle to find local qualified providers who can deliver these services (Houston, 2014b; Houston, Munoz, & Bradham, 2011; Houston & Perigoe, 2010; JCIH, 2007). Similarly, adults with hearing loss may also find it challenging to enroll in aural rehabilitation services due to a lack of availability (Galvin, Case, & Houston, 2014; Montgomery & Houston, 2000). In many regions of the world, a shortage exists of hearing health care professionals (i.e., audiologists) (Swanepoel & Hall, 2010). Thus, professionals with appropriate training who can deliver (re)habilitation services to children and adults with hearing loss are not available in every community, which affects equity of access to quality in-person services. Additionally, committing to attend in-person rehabilitation is becoming increasingly difficult for many families due to distance or work-life constraints, including having time to travel to appointments (Hayes, Qu, Weston, & Baxter, 2011). It is paramount that service providers explore time and cost-effective methods, such as telerehabilitation, to offer more flexible and equitable services to all patients, especially when barriers caused by distance, lack of services, and challenging personal circumstances exist (American Speech-Language-Hearing Association [ASHA], 2005; Houston, 2014a; Theodoros, 2013).

Advances in computer and teleconferencing technology and global improvements in telecommunications and Internet connections have allowed for the expansion of (re)habilitation services via telepractice. This chapter explores the potential for comprehensive (re)habilitation services for individuals with hearing loss to be provided at a distance through models of telerehabilitation. Over a decade ago, the ASHA published position statements and technical reports that supported telepractice as an appropriate service provision option for audiologists and speech-language pathologists. These policies noted that not all patients or treatments would be appropriate for telepractice service delivery models and that the quality of telepractice services must be equivalent to those services provided face-to-face (i.e., "in-person") (ASHA, 2005).

In this chapter, barriers to patient participation in habilitation/rehabilitation services are explored, and telerehabilitation, as a service delivery model, is shown to provide greater equity of access for children and adults with hearing loss. Models of service delivery for providing auditory-verbal therapy and aural rehabilitation through telepractice are outlined. Case studies also have been included to demonstrate the diverse circumstances whereby telepractice may be utilized for aural (re)habilitation.

Why Rehabilitation Is Important

Rehabilitation is important for children and adults to achieve optimal outcomes with their hearing technology (Boothroyd, 2007; Moeller, 2010; Tye-Murray, 2009; Yoshinaga-Itano et al., 1998). The need for rehabilitation is not governed by the age or developmental stage of a person receiving hearing technology. The length and duration of engagement in a rehabilitation program will vary depending on the specific goals of the client/family. Appropriate counseling at the time of fitting the hearing technology is essential to ensure realistic expectations are established about outcomes and to obtain the client's commitment to the rehabilitation process (Saunders, Lewis, & Forsline, 2009; Soman & Tharpe, 2012). Because hearing loss affects each member of the family in some way, clinical experience indicates the importance of a support person for both the pediatric and adult populations to assist and guide the individual with hearing loss throughout the rehabilitation process (Towey, 2013). In the pediatric population, this person is likely to be a parent or caregiver. In the adult population, it is important that the client chooses someone who is trusted and able to assist with aural rehabilitation. This person also will provide emotional support. Without a support person, the journey from fitting to the functional use of hearing technology may be more challenging. Professionals providing rehabilitation services for children and adults with hearing loss need to work closely with audiologists to ensure optimal amplification and benefit of a person's hearing technology (Estabrooks et al., 2014). Without optimal amplification, rehabilitation will not achieve the best outcomes for listening and spoken language (Cole & Flexer, 2011).

In the pediatric population, several research studies have reported outcomes of optimal amplification and intervention using a listening and spoken language approach with children with hearing loss. When children with hearing loss are identified early, fitted with appropriate hearing technology, and provided with family-centered early intervention services from properly trained professionals, most are able to progress at age-appropriate rates (Kennedy et al., 2006; Moeller, 2000; Yoshinaga-Itano et al., 1998). More positive outcomes are associated with early identification and rehabilitation, including better language, speech, and social-emotional development than later-identified children; more typical rates of cognitive development; and lower parental stress as the child acquires language and increases communication (Dornan, Hickson, Murdoch, Houston, & Constantinescu, 2010; Geers, 2006; Niparko et al., 2010; Yoshinaga-Itano & Gravel, 2001).

Rehabilitation for adults with hearing loss is often referred to as aural rehabilitation and differs from the developmental approach used with children. Rehabilitation in the adult population targets optimizing a patient's participation in life activities and alleviating difficulties caused as a result of hearing loss (Boothroyd, 2007; Estabrooks et al., 2014; Gagne, 2000; Tye-Murray, 2009). It is essential to actively involve adult patients when planning rehabilitation sessions to ensure their rehabilitation aligns with their personal goals (Estabrooks et al., 2014; McConkey Robbins, 2009). Rehabilitation that does not interest an adult or does not target functional abilities may result in poor attendance for sessions, reduced motivation, and noncompliance with using hearing technology. However, coupling the use of advanced hearing technology with aural rehabilitation services delivered by well-trained professionals can achieve improvement in auditory processing and comprehension (Houston, 2014b).

Terminology and Definitions: Telerehabilitation

Practitioners providing services to children and adults with hearing loss use a range of terms to describe the services that are delivered. Likewise, when these services are delivered using telecommunication technology via the Internet, additional terms are applied. The following list provides definitions of common terms practitioners use when engaged in aural (re)habilitation and telepractice/telerehabilitation.

- Aural habilitation: A term typically used to describe services provided to children with hearing loss, Tye-Murray (2015) defines it as "intervention for persons who have not developed and who are currently acquiring listening, speech, and language skills."
- Aural rehabilitation: Intervention aimed at minimizing and alleviating the communication difficulties associated with hearing loss (Tye-Murray, 2015), typically used to describe services provided to adults with hearing loss.
- Auditory-verbal therapy (AVT): AVT is the application and management of hearing technology, in conjunction with specific strategies, techniques, and conditions, which promote optimal acquisition of spoken language primarily through individuals listening to the sounds of their own voices, the voices of others, and all sounds of life. Listening and spoken language become a major force in nurturing the development of the child's personal, social, and academic life. When AVT is carried out with the necessary thoughtfulness, expertise, guidance, and love, most of these children develop excellent conversational competence (Estabrooks, 2012). Certified professionals in this approach are identified as listening and spoken language

specialists (LSLS), auditory-verbal therapists (Cert. AVTs), or auditory-verbal educators (Cert. AVEds).

■ Service provider/clinician/(re)habilitationist: The professional delivering intervention, habilitation, or rehabilitation services to children and adults with hearing loss. These practitioners usually have training in speech-language pathology, audiology, or education of the deaf. However, professionals from other disciplines also may be included in a continuum of services depending on the communication needs of the individual with hearing loss.

■ Client (adult/pediatric)/patient: The individual with hearing loss, either a child or adult, who is receiving services.

■ Parent/caregiver: Parents of the child with hearing loss who are the decision makers and participants in the intervention or habilitation of the child with hearing loss. In some situations, caregivers may be other family members (e.g., grandparents, aunts, uncles, etc.), nannies or au pairs, godparents, foster parents, or other significant individuals in the child's life. For adults with hearing loss, a caregiver could be a spouse, an adult child who is now providing care, a neighbor, friend, or other family member.

■ Support personnel/eHelper: Paraprofessionals who assist in the delivery of services, often at the remote site when providing telepractice services.

■ Cochlear implant mapping: Performed by a cochlear implant audiologist, this is the process of programming the speech processor, which produces a MAP. The cochlear implant recipient's MAP specifies the threshold, suprathreshold, and frequency by which the speech processor of a cochlear implant processes the speech signal and delivers it in electrical form to the electrodes in the electrode array (Tye-Murray, 2015) that is inserted into the cochlea. The term *programming* is also used to describe this process.

■ Telepractice: ASHA (2005) defines telepractice as "the application of telecommunications technology to deliver professional services at a distance by linking clinician to client, or clinician to clinician for assessment, intervention, and/or consultation." *Telepractitioner* is a term used to describe those professionals who provide services through telepractice service delivery models.

■ Telerehabilitation: These are services provided by rehabilitation practitioners, such as audiologists, occupational therapists, speech-language pathologists, physical therapists, and related disciplines. The services can incorporate intervention planning, implementation, follow-up consultation, and education (Cason, 2009). Telerehabilitation is generally characterized by repetitive service encounters over a long period of time (Brienza & McCue, 2013).

□ Categories of telerehabilitation (Brienza & McCue, 2013):

- Teleconsultation—involves the use of interactive videoconferencing between a client or local provider and a remote rehabilitationist to gain access to specialized services and expertise

- Telehomecare—involves the coordination of a rehabilitation service from various providers to the client's home (clinician may be a nurse, technician, or related practitioner)

- Teletherapy—a model of telerehabilitation whereby the client conducts therapeutic activities in the home that follows a therapy protocol managed remotely by a habilitationist

- Telemonitoring—involves client utilization of unobtrusive monitoring or assessment technology that is set up and managed by a rehabilitation provider

For the purposes of this chapter, the authors will refer to the intervention, aural (re)habilitation, or auditory-verbal therapy provided to children and adults with hearing loss via telepractice as *telerehabilitation*.

Barriers That Impact Rehabilitation Program Participation

There are a number of factors that may present as barriers to a family's or client's participation in a rehabilitation program. Some of these are individual-specific factors that may affect either the caregiver or client directly and can include grief (e.g., associated with the diagnosis of hearing loss), expectations, stress and coping strategies, and motivation or commitment to improving and making progress in functional outcomes (Fadda, 2011). Other factors that may impact participation in a rehabilitation program include availability to attend appointments around other work or family commitments (Theodoros, 2013), learning style of the caregiver or client, and socioeconomic factors that impact ability to afford even relatively small expenses involved in attendance (e.g., transportation, parking, resources, and equipment).

Ease and equity of access to service providers is a major factor for many clients, particularly those living in rural and remote locations. As the majority of specialized services are located in metropolitan areas, rural and remote clients do not have the same access to specialist care as those living in metropolitan areas (Cason, 2009; Loane & Wootton, 200: Moffatt & Eley, 2010).

The amount of travel time involved in attending appointments can negatively impact the client's participation in the program due to fatigue or frustration from traveling. As well, the parents or caregivers may experience stress caused by the need for time away from work and other family members. These situations are often exacerbated for very young and elderly clients. Parking and transportation difficulties can also be barriers (Schmeler, Schein, McCue, & Betz, 2008). The costs involved in traveling longer distances (e.g., fuel, parking, meals, flight, and hotel accommodations) can be prohibitive in some circumstances and challenging at best in others. The additional costs associated with time away from work and the potential loss of income can add significant challenges for some clients and/or families. Long-term management of clients with chronic diseases can be difficult to sustain through the face-to-face (i.e., in-person) service delivery model (Theodoros, 2013). Repeat or frequent travel requirements increase the time and cost burden for many clients and families, which may make ongoing participation in a center-based program prohibitive. Lack of consistent participation and follow-through with rehabilitation services will affect the client's long-term communication outcomes.

Although the issues relating to distance and travel for families in rural and remote areas are particularly problematic, it is also important to note that geographical proximity to specialized services is also likely to be a potential barrier to timely and appropriate treatment for clients with hearing loss, even in major metropolitan areas (Lai, Serraglio, & Martin, 2014). For example, a family with a child with hearing loss may have to take city buses and the subway to reach the service provider. Even when the family lives in the city, transportation from home to the center may be an arduous task. Adults with hearing loss, especially those who are elderly, may no longer drive themselves to appointments, or due to other health conditions, they may not have the mobility to leave their homes. A client's participation in a rehabilitation program also can be affected by the service provider's availability for appointments, flexibility in meeting client needs, workload, and experience.

Some of the barriers to participation in rehabilitation programs that have been outlined are likely to be the same for clients, regardless of their proximity to service providers or the service delivery model utilized. However, some are unique to clients living in rural or remote areas or who have reduced access to in-person service delivery models for mobility or medical reasons. These barriers can be largely overcome with an effective telerehabilitation program. Telerehabilitation, therefore, has the ability to meet the communication needs of clients in rural and remote areas (Cason, 2009) as well as other clients in similarly unique or challenging circumstances.

How Can Telepractice Help?

Telepractice enables customized rehabilitation service to all clients, regardless of their geographic location. If clients have a high-speed Internet connection (i.e., broadband) in their home, educational setting, or workplace and utilize off-the-shelf technology (e.g., desktop computer or laptop, webcam, microphone and speakers), they have the ability to participate in telerehabilitation. This minimizes the need for frequent family travel, which reduces associated costs, time, and other stressors (Loane & Wootton, 2001).

Advances in telecommunication technology and increasing access to Internet services worldwide have enabled more clients access to appropriate telehealth services from their living and learning environments (Simpson, 2013). Consumer familiarity with technology and increased client expectations about the availability of online services drive growth and greater demand for telerehabilitation (Heinzelmann, Lugn, & Kvedar, 2005; Simpson, 2013).

Delivering services in the community, such as direct services to the home or school, is considered best practice in most areas of rehabilitation (McCue, Fairman, & Pramuka, 2010). A "natural environment" model of telerehabilitation is supported in both behavioral therapy and vocational rehabilitation literature (Brienza & McCue, 2013). For both young children and adults with hearing loss, the ability to provide telerehabilitation services in the home setting is highly desirable and offers several advantages:

- parents and caregivers do not have to travel, saving time and other resources;
- adults with hearing loss may have mobility issues (i.e., unable to walk, uses a walker, or a wheelchair) or no longer drive;
- children are more comfortable, because they are in their own home with their parents and using familiar toys;
- adults may also be more comfortable receiving services in their own homes;
- the setting is the natural environment, and carryover of targeted communication goals and objectives into the child's or adult's daily routines can be easier;
- parents can practice new strategies for listening, speech, or language and be coached by well-trained practitioners, and similarly, adults can be coached directly by the service providers;
- for children with hearing loss, their siblings, when appropriate, can be integrated into the sessions more easily or be occupied and supervised;
- the adult's spouse, caregiver, or adult children can be included in the sessions, and they can learn strategies that can facilitate improved communication with the adult with hearing loss;
- for the child, other family members or caregivers, such as grandparents or nannies, may find it easier to participate in the sessions;

- sessions in the home offer greater convenience for families as they can more readily fit in sessions around other appointments and work schedules;
- children and adults with hearing loss who have minor illnesses or have mobility challenges can still have productive sessions; and
- in most cases, telerehabilitation sessions result in fewer cancellations, which allows for more timely and consistent intervention over time and results in more desired developmental and/or communicative outcomes (Houston, Behl, & Walters, 2013).

Clients who do not have high-speed or broadband Internet services in the home or have insufficient technology may have access to dedicated teleconferencing systems or computers at a neighbor's house, community health/education center, or local library. This enables those families or adults to participate in telerehabilitation. Conducting sessions utilizing one of these alternate locations can provide the additional benefit of including in the rehabilitation sessions other clinicians or support staff involved in the care of the client (e.g., caregivers, teachers, teacher aides, allied health professionals). By doing so, this may also provide indirect professional training benefits to those involved in the client's care (Loane & Wootton, 2001) and facilitate more collaborative case management and interprofessional care of the client (Heinzelmann et al., 2005).

As telerehabilitation depends less on location and time than face-to-face (i.e., in-person) models of care (Heinzelmann et al., 2005), it can provide additional flexibility in scheduling appointments. Client availability to participate is likely to be greater than if required to find time to travel to attend sessions. Service providers' availability may also be greater as a result of providing telerehabilitation services, as travel time to visit clients in rural and remote areas is greatly reduced.

Telerehabilitation enables the therapist greater flexibility to modify the sequencing, timing, and intensity of rehabilitation (Theodoros, 2013; Towey, 2013; Winters & Winters, 2004) and can offer clients living in rural or remote locations as well as metropolitan locations optimized service delivery approaches. That is, some clients may benefit from a hybrid approach whereby a portion of their services may be delivered in person within a clinic or center, while other services may be provided to them at a distance through telerehabilitation.

Clients and their families may be required to learn how to use new technology to participate in telerehabilitation sessions; however, the increase in most individuals' comfort using a notebook or tablet computer for Web conferencing (e.g., FaceTime, Skype, ooVoo, Google Hangouts, Zoom, GoToMeeting, Cisco WebEx, etc.) has ensured that specific training is needed less and less as time goes on. Where training is required, it is important to take into account the learning styles of those acquiring new skills—the client, family member, caregiver, or support personnel—to ensure a more successful and comfortable transition to telerehabilitation. Some clients may take longer to adjust to telerehabilitation than others, but with careful planning, preparation, and adequate guidance and coaching, most are able to effectively participate. In other cases, telerehabilitation may be more successful compared to center-based or in-person sessions. For example, the coaching of families at a distance requires more direct involvement of the parents, spouse, or other caregivers. Telerehabilitation places the parent or support person in the "driver's seat" (Blaiser, Behl, Callow-Heusser, & Guthrie, 2013; Houston, 2014a), and they are required to actively participate in the session. The professional, who is located at a distant center or other facility, fulfills the role of coach. Additionally, some clients grow to prefer this method of service delivery to traditional face-to-face (i.e., in person) service delivery for the skill development and flexibility that is provides.

During telerehabilitation sessions, rapport can be established and maintained because the clinician and client are able to see and hear each other (Blaiser et al., 2013; Houston, 2014a; Loane & Wootton, 2001). Service providers who have the appropriate training and experience are able to counsel parents, families, or other caregivers as they would during in-person sessions. They are able to guide and coach parents and caregivers in the use of new strategies and techniques to enhance communication with the family member with hearing loss.

For professionals, obtaining the skills to provide rehabilitation through a telepractice service delivery model is important for ensuring successful outcomes (Cason, 2009; Jarvis- Selinger, Chan, Payne, Plohman, & Ho, 2008; Towey, 2013). Likewise, the education, training, and experience of service providers also will impact the quality of aural (re)habilitation, regardless of service delivery method. Clinicians who have clinical experience providing face-to-face services are likely to have most of the foundational skills and expertise necessary for providing services via telepractice. However, additional training and ongoing support may be required to ensure adaption to delivering services remotely (Houston, 2014a; Jarvis-Selinger et al., 2008; Loane & Wootton, 2001). Some of the following skills should be acquired:

- use of telecommunications and computer technology and troubleshooting;
- modification of service delivery to explain how to carry out skills rather than personally demonstrating skills (Cason, 2009); and
- observation of performance and elicitation of feedback from parents and caregivers regarding client performance.

A well-managed and executed telerehabilitation program should deliver services and client outcomes that are equivalent to those achieved in traditional face-to-face models. Service providers delivering telerehabilitation also should have confidence in the suitability and sustainability of such programs (Jarvis-Selinger et al., 2008). Telepractice is an effective service delivery model for the provision of rehabilitation in clients with hearing loss. However, it is important to understand that when clinical judgment is impacted by this mode of service delivery, in-person sessions or consultations can be arranged in place of, or in addition to, telerehabilitation sessions. Ultimately, the needs of the client should dictate the service delivery model—whether it is telerehabilitation, traditional in-person sessions, or a combination of the two (i.e., a hybrid approach).

How Do You Deliver Rehabilitation Services via Telepractice?

Over the past decade, audiologists and speech-language pathologists have increasingly adopted models of telepractice to provide comprehensive diagnostic and treatment services to their patients (Houston, 2014a; Kumar & Cohn, 2013). As these services continue to expand to a range of populations, a growing number of practitioners are choosing to provide telerehabilitation services to children and adults with hearing loss, often achieving outcomes that rival in-person service delivery (Constantinescu, 2012; Constantinescu et al., 2014; Galvan et al., 2014; Houston, 2014b; Stedler-Brown, 2012). Two such programs that have developed innovative telerehabilitation programs are the Hear and Say Centre in Brisbane, Australia, and the Telepractice and eLearning Laboratory (TeLL), which is housed in the School of Speech-Language Pathology and Audiology at the University of Akron in Akron, Ohio.

The Hear and Say Centre

The Hear and Say Centre provides AVT (i.e., listening and spoken language) early intervention, has school support services for children and adolescents with hearing loss, and has a Hearing Implant Program that provides candidacy assessment and postimplant clinical care and assessments for eligible individuals with hearing loss. Hear and Say has six centers throughout Queensland that provide traditional in-person services and an "eAuditory-Verbal Therapy" (eAVT) telepractice program, which launched in 1998 to provide habilitation services to families living in rural and remote locations throughout Queensland. The telepractice program has grown significantly, and its services have more recently been extended to some families living in metropolitan areas that find it more appropriate to access home-based services. Telerehabilitation has also been utilized to serve adolescent and adult implant recipients in the Hear and Say rehabilitation program.

AVT in early intervention is typically a parent-focused program: In an in-person session, an auditory-verbal therapist will design activities to address the listening and spoken language goals of the child. During the session, the therapist models how to carry out the activity and then hands over the activity to the parent. The therapist's role shifts to that of coach, and the therapist then guides the parents in how to interact with their child to maximize listening and spoken language.

When conducting AVT via telepractice, the therapist should carefully explain to a parent exactly how to prepare for, introduce, and carry out an activity with his or her child (in the absence of being able to model directly with the child first). At the Hear and Say Centre, this is achieved through conducting planning sessions via Web conferencing with a parent one week and then observing, guiding, and coaching the parent in delivering these activities with their child via Web conferencing the following week. The therapist documents the child's performance during a session, and the parent and therapist discuss the child's progress (Figures 7–1 and 7–2).

Families in the Hear and Say Centre's early intervention telerehabiltiation program are provided with age-appropriate lesson boxes that contain toys, puzzles, books, games, and other resources that can be utilized in lessons. Families are loaned these resources for a period of time, which are then returned and replaced with another lesson box. Therapists are able to see the contents of the box on an electronic catalogue system, which helps with preparation and planning for lessons. Alternatively,

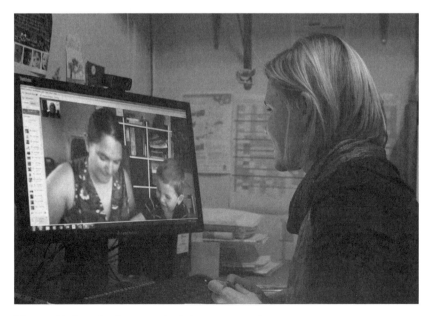

Figure 7–1. eAuditory-verbal therapy session.

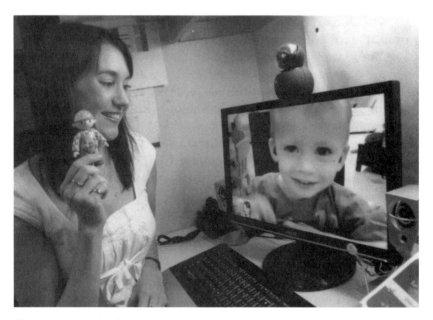

Figure 7–2. eAuditory-verbal therapy session.

inventories of home resources, crafts, and other items may be utilized to plan activities for the sessions (Figure 7–3).

Any additional consultations (e.g., behavior management, occupational therapy, or social work support) can be provided via telepractice, either built into existing sessions or in place of typical telerehabilitation sessions. Clients with cochlear implants are provided with telemapping services when appropriate. Families enrolled in Hear and Say's telepractice program receive in-person contact approximately four times each year in addition to weekly Web conferencing sessions. Twice each year, their auditory-verbal therapist travels to their home to conduct home visits as well as inclusive educational setting visits for school-age children (providing consultation and advice on working with children with hearing loss). Families also attend the Hear and Say Centre to participate in speech and language assessments, social skills groups, parent education sessions, and group/individual lessons. Waite et al. (Waite, Cahill, Theodoros, Busuttin, & Russell, 2006; Waite, Theodoros, Russell, & Cahill, 2010) con-

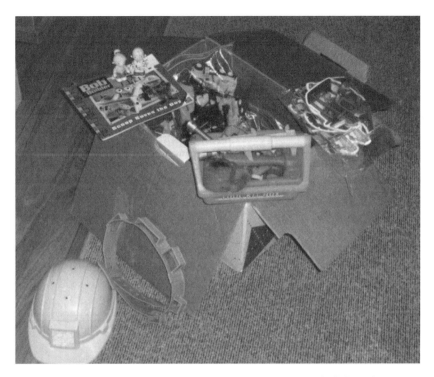

Figure 7–3. Example of a resource box, based on a building theme.

ducted a number of validation studies on completing standardized speech and language assessments via telepractice; however, further research is required in order for this to become part of routine clinical practice.

Hear and Say has an "all of life" hearing implant program; this means that adolescent and adult clients also receive services. Telepractice has allowed a more flexible approach to service delivery for each client in an effort to meet specific communication goals and individual needs. Offering telerehabilitation has enabled more consistent and frequent services for many clients who are unable to attend in-person sessions due to distance or hectic work schedules. Telerehabilitation has allowed for a comprehensive block of time devoted to improving their communication skills. For adolescents and adults, telerehabilitation sessions differ slightly from eAuditory-verbal therapy services in the early intervention program. The client and therapist will connect through Web conferencing and cover the following points:

- discuss the progress they have made since their last session,
- discuss any barriers or problems that have presented to them since the last session,
- discuss the next steps/goals for improving their listening skills,
- discuss activities to practice and target in order to develop those skills, and
- discuss home follow-up.

After the telerehabilitation session concludes, an email is sent to the client and support person to follow up on the next goals. This cycle of support and rehabilitation continues through telerehabilitation until the client and therapist agree that they have reached the established communication goals and maximized the listening potential of the client.

Telepractice and eLearning Laboratory (TeLL): The University of Akron

To increase the availability of auditory-verbal (i.e., listening and spoken language) intervention for children with hearing loss and their families and adult aural rehabilitation services in Ohio, the Telepractice and eLearning Laboratory (TeLL) was established in the Audiology and Speech Center, which is the primary on-campus clinical training facility for the School of Speech-Language Pathology and Audiology at The University of Akron. In addition to direct service provision, the development of the TeLL also has allowed for ongoing data collection in the study of telepractice service delivery models and has served as an intensive practicum experience for graduate students in speech-language pathology.

Currently, the TeLL is providing auditory-verbal intervention to infants, toddlers, preschoolers, and school-age children with hearing loss and their families. These children and their families are following a listening and spoken language approach that is supported by the principles of auditory-verbal practice

(Estabrooks, 2012). Likewise, a growing number of adults with hearing loss, whether they are utilizing digital hearing aids or cochlear implants, are receiving aural rehabilitation services through a telepractice service delivery model.

Families of children with hearing loss and adults who require comprehensive aural rehabilitation services experience similar frustrations when attempting to secure appropriate services, often making both groups appropriate candidates for telepractice services. Although not an exhaustive list, as noted in Houston (2014a), individuals may turn to telepractice service delivery models for a variety of reasons, especially when

- consumers who are more "tech friendly" demand or prefer telepractice or related services;
- a shortage of qualified clinicians, interventions, treatment approaches, or clinical services exist in their community;
- travel constraints or a lack of transportation prohibit obtaining appropriate services;
- mobility issues prevent or restrict leaving the home;
- chronic medical or other health issues complicate receiving traditional in-person services;
- superior services may be delivered through telepractice —rather than through in-person, center-based services;
- telepractice services received in the patient's home offer more flexibility of scheduling, resulting in fewer cancelations and more consistent intervention and treatment;
- telepractice services may prove to be more cost-effective and efficient in meeting the patient's needs;
- telepractice services delivered in the home provide a more functional, natural environment for intervention and treatment; and
- parents and other family members benefit from coaching strategies that will help the patient, which results in improved long-term treatment outcomes.

TeLL: Serving Children With Hearing Loss and Their Families

The practice of AVT requires full parent participation in each session, and as described above, the parent is the main "consumer" of the intervention. That is, the trained professional provides coaching and guidance to ensure that the parent becomes the primary facilitator of listening and spoken language for the child with hearing loss. As the parent's knowledge and skills increase, the child's auditory functioning and use of spoken language also improve. Telepractice remains a valuable service delivery tool that can connect parents of children with hearing loss who have chosen an auditory-verbal approach to qualified practitioners.

Through the TeLL, families receive weekly auditory-verbal telepractice sessions. Because the University of Akron has two listening and spoken language specialists and certified auditory-verbal therapists (LSLS Cert. AVTs) on faculty, a commitment exists to provide comprehensive listening and spoken language services to children with hearing loss and their families. Furthermore, the School of Speech-Language Pathology and Audiology remains one of only a few university training programs that incorporates auditory-verbal content in its courses and provides clinical practicum experiences in support of listening and spoken language outcomes for children with hearing loss. In fact, the School of Speech-Language Pathology and Audiology at the University of Akron, in collaboration with The University of Toledo, are two of a limited number of university training programs that have funding from the U.S. Department of Education that support personnel preparation in the area of listening and spoken language for children with hearing loss. The Graduate Studies Consortium in Listening and Spoken Language was formed between these two universities to provide coursework, practica, and field-based experiences to graduate students completing this training. Thus, through the TeLL, graduate students in speech-language pathology not only learn how to deliver effective auditory-verbal sessions but also learn how to provide these services through a telepractice model as well as traditional, in-person center-based sessions (Figure 7–4).

Currently, the TeLL is housed in a converted treatment room in the Audiology and Speech Center. A Dell Optiplex 9010 desktop computer is connected to a 32-inch Toshiba flat-screen television that is used as a monitor. The Phoenix USB Speakerphone serves as an integrated audio microphone and speaker. The webcam is a Logitech Orbit AF Quickcam. Because the University of Akron utilizes WebEx as its primary distance learn-

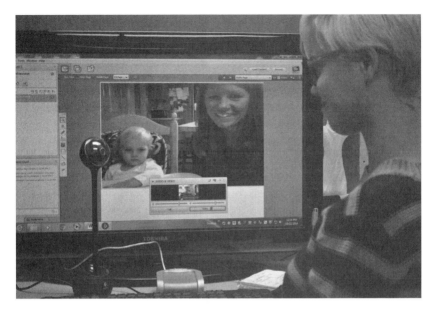

Figure 7–4. Auditory-verbal telepractice session.

ing software, the same software is used for all telepractice sessions. Graduate students and faculty receive guided training on the use of the software and preferred practices for delivering telepractice services prior to any treatment. Privacy, confidentiality, and appropriate software encryption are carefully monitored and maintained. Once treatment is initiated with patients, graduate students continue to be closely supervised by experienced faculty.

Referrals of families with children with hearing loss are received primarily from pediatric audiologists, otolaryngology/otology practices, cochlear implant programs, speech-language pathologists, other parents of children with hearing loss, and through informal "word-of-mouth" connections. Typically, once a referral is received, the following process occurs:

1. a preliminary case history is gathered, usually over the telephone;
2. the child (and family) is scheduled for a comprehensive, in-person speech and language evaluation at the Audiology and Speech Center;

3. the diagnostic assessment is completed evaluating functional hearing/speech perception with the child's hearing technology (e.g., digital hearing aids, cochlear implants, and/or assistive listening device), speech production, receptive and expressive language, and oral-motor development (note: other assessment areas may be added—depending on the needs of the child);

4. once the assessment is completed, a determination is made regarding the use of service delivery models: telepractice or in-person, center-based intervention;

5. if telepractice is recommended, the parents will complete a short questionnaire about the type of computer equipment they have in their home or where they may have access to a computer with the necessary components (webcam, audio speakers, and microphone) as well as a broadband Internet connection;

   a. if it is determined that the parents have the necessary computer equipment available to them, a session will be scheduled to "test" the connection and their comfort with the telepractice session; and

   b. finally, if the connection is successful and the parents feel comfortable with WebEx, the first formal telepractice session is then scheduled.

On occasion, a family who initially seemed to be excellent candidates for telepractice may have difficulty with the service delivery model. That is, there may be technological challenges that emerge or, after beginning services, the parents may find themselves struggling to incorporate the listening and spoken language strategies that are demonstrated through telepractice. Similarly, other behavioral or learning needs may be identified in the child that require additional services that cannot be addressed through telepractice. In these rare cases, a hybrid model of service delivery may be implemented whereby the family may come to the Audiology and Speech Center for in-person, center-based services on alternating weeks while continuing to gain confidence with telepractice. Over time, the in-person sessions may be reduced as the family transitions to receiving all of the treatment services through telepractice. Ultimately, the first priority is to ensure that telepractice can provide an equivalent level of service delivery and that the communication needs of the child (and family) are being met.

Although an occasional family may require a hybrid model of telepractice, most do not and usually adapt very quickly. After the child has completed the initial speech and language assessment and the family's computer technology is tested (as outlined above), regular telepractice sessions are scheduled. Prior to each weekly 60-minute session, the family receives a lesson plan and materials through email that were developed to meet the child's current goals in speech, language, and listening. Many of the materials, such as colorful scenes to foster language use, can be printed in the home and used during the therapy session in the form of PowerPoint files. The email will also contain a Web link that, once clicked, will launch Cisco WebEx. The parents enter the "virtual classroom" and can see these materials as images on their computer screen.

Because Cisco WebEx provides teleconferencing—complete audio and video in real time—each session begins with a discussion of the speech, language, and listening goals targeted during the prior session. The discussion also includes how the parent has integrated previously demonstrated communication strategies into the child's daily routines. The faculty member, graduate students, and parent discuss any new communication behaviors that might be relevant to the child's progress, such as new or emerging speech sounds, words, or listening behaviors that have been noticed. Once these updates have occurred, the faculty member and graduate students introduce the goals for that day's session, explaining the desired speech, language, listening, and interactive behaviors.

After discussing the materials and activities for the session, the faculty member and/or graduate students demonstrate the activity before asking the parent to engage the child. The parent repeats the activity while the faculty member and graduate students observe. At this point in the session, the practitioner's role shifts to that of a coach. The faculty member and/or graduate student provides positive reinforcement and constructive feedback to the parent based on how the activity was implemented and how the communication strategies that promote listening and spoken language are applied. This same scenario is repeated as one activity ends and a new activity is initiated. Throughout the session, the parent, the faculty member, and graduate students closely monitor the child's attention level and communication targets.

Following the session, the parent is given ample opportunity to discuss any concerns about the child's progress, to ask questions about short- or long-term communication goals, or to seek input about troubleshooting the child's hearing technology (e.g., digital hearing aids and/or cochlear implants, FM systems). The faculty member and graduate students summarize the goals and facilitation strategies that were modeled and practiced during the session. Based on the child's performance and developmental level, new or additional communication goals are discussed that will be targeted in the home the following week.

TeLL: Adult Aural Rehabilitation

As described by Tye-Murray (2009), aural rehabilitation is aimed at restoring or optimizing a patient's participation in activities that have been limited as a result of hearing loss and also may be aimed at benefiting communication partners who engage in activities that include persons with hearing loss. The goals of aural rehabilitation are to alleviate the difficulties related to hearing loss and minimize its consequences (Gagne, 2000; Tye-Murray, 2009). Although these goals are clear, patients with hearing loss may struggle to identify aural rehabilitation services in their community and may be either unserved or underserved (Tye-Murray, 2009). Reasons for this occurring include a dearth of outreach and immediate or extended support services, the attitudes of service delivery personnel, the lack of reimbursement policies for aural rehabilitation, and communication or environmental barriers (Tye-Murray, 2009). Thus, for adults with hearing loss who are utilizing a range of hearing technology (e.g., digital hearing aids, cochlear implants, assistive listening devices), telepractice service delivery models—like those provided through the TeLL—may be a viable means of connecting patients with qualified speech-language pathologists and audiologists who can provide aural rehabilitation.

Like many of the pediatric patients, adults with hearing loss are referred from several sources, including primary care physicians, audiologists, speech-language pathologists, cochlear implant centers, and word of mouth from other individuals with hearing loss. Typically, once an adult referral is received, a similar diagnostic and treatment process occurs:

1. a preliminary case history is gathered, usually over the telephone with the adult (if the adult has enough hearing acuity to use the telephone) or with the patient's spouse or adult children who may be assisting with securing aural rehabilitation services;
2. the adult (and spouse and adult children) is scheduled for a comprehensive communication evaluation at the Audiology and Speech Center that assesses functional speech perception with his or her hearing technology (e.g., digital hearing aids, cochlear implants, and/ or assistive listening device), speech production, and language (as well as other communication areas, if needed);
3. once the assessment is completed, a determination is made regarding the use of service delivery models: telepractice or in-person, center-based intervention;
4. if telepractice is recommended, the adult (or spouse and family) will complete a short questionnaire about the type of computer equipment he or she has in the home or where he or she may have access to a computer with the necessary components (webcam, audio speakers, and microphone) as well as a broadband Internet connection;
   a. if it is determined that the adult has the necessary computer equipment available, a session will be scheduled to test the connection and his or her comfort with the telepractice session; and
   b. finally, if the connection is successful and the adult (and spouse) feels comfortable with the Collaborate software, the first formal telepractice session is then scheduled.

For adult patients receiving services through the TeLL, each session is focused on the individual's communication needs in the areas of auditory processing and overall conversational competence. Using Cisco WebEx, the adult logs into the virtual classroom from his or her home computer and Internet connection, and the faculty member and graduate students are able to interact directly with the patient. The session typically begins with a discussion of how the patient has performed over the past week since the previous session. Any noticeable changes in the patient's communication—either positive or negative—are recorded in his or her file. Then, a discussion of the current session's goals and activities occurs. Typically, most patients have goals that target auditory discrimination and identification tasks at the phoneme and word levels. That is, these activities provide "bottom-up" auditory skills that are essential for making fine discrimination of speech information. As well, most patients have a communication partner that participates in every session, such as his or her spouse or grown (adult) children who are now assisting in the rehabilitation process or assuming a larger caretaking role for the parent.

Conversely, the patient also will have activities that target "top-down" activities that incorporate functional language and conversational skills. Throughout the session, the faculty member and graduate students are giving directions, asking questions, and commenting on the patient's performance. Even when formal top-down strategies are not being targeted directly, these skills are being practiced indirectly. For each adult patient, top-down language activities and conversations are tailored to meet his or her specific needs. That is, patients may share vocabulary or conversational phrases from their profession or work setting, and those are incorporated into each session. Additionally, many adults may also struggle with specific listening situations within the community, such as attending a worship service, a restaurant, a local business, or the gym. Context-specific phrases and vocabulary from these situations are also practiced within the telepractice session.

Counseling is an essential component of most telepractice sessions with adults receiving aural rehabilitation. For some adults, the focus may be on assisting them to have realistic expectations about their level of progress after receiving a cochlear implant(s). For others, counseling may address strategies to stay motivated to use their hearing technology, to reenter the workforce, or to practice newly acquired skills—especially if the hearing loss has had a sudden onset. As well, the counseling paradigm is not limited to or focused solely on the patient. The patient's hearing loss has affected the spouse and other family members. Their challenges and successes as well as hopes and fears should be addressed appropriately. And finally, many adults respond positively when interacting with other adults who have shared similar life experiences. For this reason, patients receiving services through the TeLL also attend a monthly support group that provides informational and educational counseling as well as opportunities to converse with others with hearing loss. Spouses and family members also attend and have dedicated time in their own support group.

Case Study 1

Alex is a 4-year-old female who began a listening and spoken language (AVT) early intervention program via telepractice immediately after being diagnosed at birth with a bilateral moderate-to-moderately severe sensorineural hearing loss. Alex and her family reside interstate at approximately 425 miles (685 km) from her audiologist and telerehabilitationist. She wears bilateral hearing aids that require monitoring to ensure that she continues to receive adequate auditory access to all the sounds of the speech spectrum.

Alex's mother connects with the telerehabilitationist via telepractice to discuss progress and to plan lesson activities that address listening and spoken language goals. This planning session occurs 1 week prior to the lesson, which is conducted through Web conferencing the following week. Alex's mother receives a lesson plan from the therapist prior to the lesson to remind her of materials needed and goals to be addressed in the session. She carries out the activities planned and adjusts her interactions with Alex as guided by her therapist. The therapist coaches the mother to use strategies that maximize Alex's listening and spoken language skills. The mother conducts follow-up activities in the home and monitors Alex's progress between telerehabilitation sessions. Positive outcomes and/or concerns about progress are discussed with her telerehabilitationist during subsequent sessions.

Because Alex attends a local preschool program 2 days per week, some planning sessions and lessons are scheduled with Alex's mother and her teacher/itinerant support teacher.

This ensures that her listening and spoken language goals are monitored and addressed in all learning environments and also enables her parents and all professionals involved in Alex's care to collaborate regularly regarding her progress and development.

Case Study 2

Isabella is a 3.5-year-old female who receives AVT through telerehabilitation and cochlear implant mapping via teleaudiology services. Isabella and her family live 332 miles (534 km) from their audiologist and listening and spoken language specialist.

Isabella was diagnosed with hearing loss at birth. She received her hearing aids and began telerehabilitation at 6 months of age. At this time, her family lived in a rural town 215 miles (347 km) from their service providers, and telerehabilitation was the only service delivery option. They began weekly telerehabilitation through Web conferencing, which included alternating weeks of parent planning sessions and AVT sessions.

At 1.5 years of age, Isabella's hearing deteriorated, and she received bilateral cochlear implants. This initially required more trips to the metropolitan center for mapping, and she received in-person habilitation while there. At age 2, her family moved to the town where they now reside. Despite the move, Isabella and her family were able to remain engaged with the same service provider and continue their telerehabilitation support. The move to their new location also allowed them to receive teleaudiology support for cochlear implant programming. The flexibility of telerehabilitation has allowed a continuous supportive rehabilitation program and greater access to teleaudiology services. Delivering services through a telepractice model has reduced travel time and the financial commitment required to access a listening and spoken language program.

Case Study 3

Sam is a 22-year-old male who initiated rehabilitation after receiving a sequential bilateral cochlear implant. Sam resides 95 miles (150 km) from his audiologist and telepractitioner. Sam wore hearing aids after a diagnosis of bilateral severe sensorineural hearing loss at a young age and attended an AVT program. He received his first cochlear implant at 11 years of age when his hearing deteriorated. Sam's decision to receive a second (bilateral) cochlear implant was related to his education and career goals, as he wanted better hearing in noisy environments and improved telephone use. Sam's parents supported him throughout the bilateral rehabilitation process.

Sam initially attended in-person therapy after cochlear implant mapping appointments. When mapping sessions were reduced and became less frequent, the decision was made to conduct telerehabilitation sessions. Telerehabilitation reduced Sam's travel, saved time, and lessened the financial burden while still providing support and guidance to achieve his rehabilitation goals. Sam reported that he was particularly pleased with the flexibility telerehabilitation sessions allowed. He connected for one session using his laptop and mobile phone wireless hotspot while sitting in his car as he was on the way to a friend's house at the time of our appointment. Sam still receives in-person rehabilitation when he attends mapping sessions, but he is now supported using a flexible hybrid model that includes both telerehabilitation and in-person aural rehabilitation.

Case Study 4

John is a 63-year-old male who contracted meningitis at age 60 and experienced sudden and permanent hearing loss, a reduction in visual acuity, and a balance disorder. After leaving the hospital for treatment for meningitis, John was diagnosed with bilateral severe-to-profound sensorineural hearing loss in his left ear and a moderate-to-severe sensorineural hearing loss in his right ear. His vision did improve slightly, and he required a stronger prescription with his glasses. The balance issues also resolved, and he now has little to no problems with walking.

Within 3 months of leaving the hospital for treatment of the meningitis, John decided to receive a cochlear implant in his left ear, and he chose to wear a hearing aid in his right ear. Initially, John chose to attend in-person aural rehabilitation sessions in the hospital where he received his cochlear implant. He responded well to rehabilitation, but he soon sought a second opinion about his amount of progress. Because he was returning to work as an attorney, he also sought out services that were more flexible and fit into his rather hectic schedule.

For John, continuing aural rehabilitation through telerehabilitation provided greater flexibility of scheduling and proved to be more effective and efficient over time. The aural rehabilitation plan consisted of bottom-up and top-down skills and communication strategies. In the beginning, John struggled discriminating and identifying specific phonemes, syllables, and words. Aural rehabilitation lessons targeted those troublesome items, and the clinicians also included legal terminology that he also struggled to understand through audition alone. Assisting John in determining context cues that would aid in his comprehension continued to be an aural rehabilitation goal for him. Several top-down strategies also were targeted, especially those that specifically dealt with communication breakdown and repair. John often did not share that he had a hearing loss, and he would, at times, fail to acknowledge when he did not understand his communication partner. These areas of skill development were also incorporated into this aural rehabilitation plan.

Today, John continues to receive aural rehabilitation through telepractice two times each month. He remains very productive as an attorney, and he enjoys getting his listening skills "tuned up" during the sessions. Although his hearing will never return to what it was prior to contracting meningitis, John continues to refine his communication skills, and telepractice provided him access to aural rehabilitation services that have allowed him to remain socially active and professionally productive.

Telerehabilitation: A Structure to Support Interprofessional Service Provision

Children and adults with hearing loss often receive services from a range of providers, clinicians, and medical personnel. For a variety of reasons, these professionals—although well meaning —may fail to adequately communicate with each other, which can place the patient/client in the middle of a maelstrom of conflicting diagnoses, treatment protocols, and long-term prognoses. Interprofessional health care and, more specifically, interprofessional health care teams seek to focus on relationship-centered collaborations beyond the traditional core groups of physicians, nurses, and therapists; it incorporates all of the constituencies who impact patient outcomes. Working interprofessionally requires the breakdown of professional boundaries—without violating ethical standards and practices—to target the specific, individualized needs of the patient (Weiss, Tilin, & Morgan, 2014).

Multidisciplinary and interdisciplinary teams have existed in speech-language pathology and audiology for years, but working interprofessionally may be a new concept for some professionals. Telerehabilitation offers a unique framework to support interprofessional collaboration for both children and adults with hearing loss. For example, the toddler with hearing loss who receives early intervention physical therapy services in the home, participates in AVT via telepractice, and continues to be managed audiologically by the audiologist at the children's hospital, which is a 2-hour drive from the home, would benefit from these service providers being in contact regularly or even co-treating under appropriate conditions. In this situation, the telepractice session could be structured so that the auditory-verbal therapist could observe the child's physical therapy session to better understand the child's range of mobility and how to incorporate those goals into the AVT sessions. Likewise, the physical therapist, while visiting the home, could observe and participate in the AVT session to understand the child's communication goals, abilities, and limitations. At any time, the audiologist could be included in the sessions to ensure an open line of communication, to answer questions about the child's audiological management, and to exchange updates about the child's level of developmental and communication progress. Similarly, adults with hearing loss can benefit from well-coordinated interprofessional collaboration as part of their aural rehabilitation that is delivered through telepractice.

Telerehabilitation is yet to be fully utilized within audiology, and children and adults with hearing loss, as well as their families, not only will benefit from these services but also may receive improved service coordination among their providers through strong interprofessional teaming. Telerehabilitation provides a framework for more consistent interprofessional communication, coordination, and collaboration, which, in turn, will lead to greater patient satisfaction and improved intervention and rehabilitation outcomes.

Summary

Telerehabilitation (i.e., telepractice) service delivery models continue to evolve within speech-language pathology and audiology, and practitioners increasingly are utilizing distance technology to provide audiological, speech, and language services to young children with hearing loss and their families as well as adults with hearing loss. From hearing screenings and diagnostics to hearing aid fittings and cochlear implant mapping, it is apparent that audiologists are adopting models of telepractice to deliver a range of services (Swanepoel & Hall, 2010). Looking forward, it is apparent that telepractice service delivery models will likely become standards of care for families seeking early intervention and/or speech and language services for their children with hearing loss. As well, adults who are utilizing digital hearing aids and/or cochlear implants will seek aural rehabilitation services to improve their auditory processing and communicative competence. For audiologists and speech-language pathologists, telerehabilitation also offers new opportunities to collaborate interprofessionally, providing a more integrated approach to serving shared patients. Most importantly, models of telepractice provide exciting opportunities to connect with patients to provide valuable services, such as AVT and/or adult aural rehabilitation, that may not be available otherwise.

References

American Speech-Language-Hearing Association (ASHA). (2005). *Speech-language pathologists providing clinical services via telepractice: Position statement.* Retrieved May 5, 2014, from http://www.asha.org/Practice-Portal/Professional-Issues/Telepractice/

Blaiser, K. M., Behl, D., Callow-Heusser, C., & White, K. R. (2013). Measuring costs and outcomes of tele-intervention when serving families of children who are deaf/hard-of-hearing. *International Journal of Telerehabilitation, 5*(2), 3–10.

Boothroyd, A. (2007). Adult aural rehabilitation: What is it and does it work? *Trends in Amplification, 11*(2), 63–71.

Brienza, D. M., & McCue, M. (2013). Introduction to telerehabilitation. In S. Kumar & E. R. Cohn (Eds.), *Telerehabilitation* (pp. 1–11). London, UK: Springer.

Cason, J. (2009). A pilot telerehabilitation program: Delivering early intervention services to rural families. *International Journal of Telerehabilitation, 1*(1), 29–38.

Cole, E. B., & Flexer, C. (2011). *Children with hearing loss: Developing listening and talking, birth to six* (2nd ed.). San Diego, CA: Plural.

Constantinescu, G. (2012). Satisfaction with telemedicine for teaching listening and spoken language to children with hearing loss. *Journal of Telemedicine and Telecare, 18,* 267–272.

Constantinescu, G., Waite, M., Dornan, D., Rushbrooke, E., Brown, J., McGovern, J., . . . Hill, A. (2014). A pilot study of telepractice delivery for teaching listening and spoken language to children with hearing loss. *Journal of Telemedicine and Telecare, 20*(3), 135–140.

Dornan, D., Hickson, L., Murdoch, B., Houston, T., & Constantinescu, G. (2010). Is auditory-verbal therapy effective for children with hearing loss? *Volta Review, 110*(3), 361–387.

Estabrooks, W. (Ed.) (2012). *101 frequently asked questions about auditory-verbal practice.* Washington, DC: Alexander Graham Bell Association for the Deaf and Hard of Hearing.

Estabrooks, W., Houston, K. T., & MacIver-Lux, K. (2014). Therapeutic approaches following cochlear implantation. In S. B. Waltzman & J. T. Roland (Eds.), *Cochlear implants* (3rd ed.). New York, NY: Thieme Medical.

Fadda, S. (2011). Psychological aspects when counselling families who have children with cochlear implants. *The Journal of Maternal-Fetal and Neonatal Medicine, 24*(Suppl. 1), 104–106.

Gagne, J. P. (2000). What I treatment evaluation research? What is its relationship to the goals of audiological rehabilitation? Who are the stakeholders of this type of research? *Ear and Hearing, 21,* S60–S73.

Galvan, C., Case, E., & Houston, K. T. (2014). Listening and learning: Using telepractice to serve children and adults with hearing loss. *Perspectives on Telepractice, 4*(1), 11–22.

Geers, A. (2006). Factors influencing spoken language outcomes in children following early cochlear implantation. *Advanced Otorhinolaryngology, 64,* 50–65.

Hayes, A., Qu, L., Weston, R., & Baxter, J. (2011). *Families in Australia 2011: Sticking together in good and tough times.* Australian Institute of Family Studies, P1–28. Retrieved May, 30, 2014, from http://www.aifs.gov.au/institute/pubs/factssheets/2011/fw2011/fw2011.pdf

Heinzelmann, P. J., Lugn, N. E., & Kvedar, J. C. (2005). Telemedicine in the future. *Journal of Telemedicine and Telecare, 11,* 384–390.

Houston, K. T. (2014a). *Telepractice in speech-language pathology.* San Diego, CA: Plural.

Houston, K, T. (2014b). *Connecting to communicate: Using telepractice to improve outcome for children and adults with hearing loss.* ASHA SIG 18. Retrieved May 5, 2014, from http://www.asha.org/aud/Articles/Using-Telepractice-to-Improve-Outcomes-for-Children-and-Adults-With-Hearing-Loss/

Houston, K. T., Behl, D., & Walters, K. Z. (2013). Using telepractice to improve outcomes for children with hearing loss & their families. In L. R. Schmeltz (Ed.), *The NCHAM EHDI* [eBook]. Retrieved December 15 2014, from http://www.infanthearing.org/ehdi-ebook/2013_ebook/18Chapter17UsingTelepractive2013.pdf

Houston, K. T., Munoz, K. F., & Bradham, T. S. (2011). Professional development: Are we meeting the needs of state EHDI programs? *The Volta Review, 111*(2), 209–223.

Houston, K. T., & Perigoe, C. B. (Eds.). (2010). Professional preparation for listening and spoken language practitioners. *The Volta Review, 110*(2), 86–354.

Jarvis-Selinger, S., Chan, E., Payne, R., Plohman, K., & Ho, K. (2008). Clinical telehealth across the discipline: Lessons learned. *Telemedicine and e-Health, 14*(7), 720–725.

Joint Committee on Infant Hearing. (2007). Year 2007 position statement: Principles and guidelines for early hearing detection and intervention programs. *Pediatrics, 120*(4), 898–921.

Kennedy, C. R., McCann, D. C., Campbell, M. J., Law, C. M., Mullee, M., Petrou, S., . . . Stevenson, J. (2006). Language ability after early detection of permanent childhood hearing impairment. *New England Journal of Medicine, 354*(20), 2131–2141.

Kumar, S., & Cohn, E. R. (Eds.). (2013). *Telerehabilitation.* London, UK: Springer.

Lai, F. Y. X., Serraglio, C., & Martin, J. A. (2014) Examining potential barriers to early intervention access in Australian hearing impaired children. *International Journal of Pediatric Otorhinolaryngology, 78,* 507–512.

Loane, M., & Wootton, R. (2001). A review of telehealth. *Medical Principles and Practice, 10,* 163–170.

McConkey Robbins, A. (2009). Rehabilitation after cochlear implantation. In J. Niparko & G. Nager (Eds.), *Cochlear implants: Principles and practices* (pp. 270–311). Baltimore, MD: Lippincott Williams & Wilkins.

McCue, M., Fairman, A., & Pramuka, M. (2010). Enhancing quality of life through telerehabilitation. *Physical Medicine and Rehabilitation Clinics of North America, 21*(1), 195–205.

Moeller, M. P. (2000). Early intervention and language development in children who are deaf and hard of hearing. *Pediatrics, 106*, E43.

Moffatt, J. J., & Eley, D. S. (2010). The reported benefits of telehealth for rural Australians. *Australian Health Review, 34*, 276–281.

Montgomery, A. A., & Houston, K. T. (2000). Management of the hearing-impaired adult. In J. Alpiner & P. McCarthy (Eds.), *Rehabilitative audiology: Children and adults* (3rd ed.). Baltimore, MD: Williams & Wilkins.

Niparko, J. K., Tobey, E. A., Thal, D. J., Eisenberg, L. S., Nae-Yuh, W., Quittner, A. L., & Fink, N. E. (2010). Spoken language development in children following cochlear implantation. *JAMA: Journal of the American Medical Association, 303*(15), 1498–1506.

Saunders, G. H., Lewis, M. S., & Forsline, A. (2009). Expectations, prefitting counseling, and hearing aid outcome. *Journal of the American Academy of Audiology, 20*(5), 320–334.

Schmeler, M. R., Schein, R. M., McCue, M., & Betz, K. (2008, Fall). Telerehabilitation clinical and vocational applications for assistive technology: Research, opportunities, and challenges. *International Journal of Telerehabilitation*, pp. 12–24.

Simpson, J. (2013). Challenges and trends driving telerehabilitation. In S. Kumar & E. R. Cohn (Eds.), *Telerehabilitation* (pp. 13–27). London, UK: Springer.

Soman, U. G., & Tharpe, A. M. (2012). Rehabilitation and educational considerations for children with cochlear implants. *Otolaryngologic Clinics of North America, 45*(1), 141–153.

Stedler-Brown, A. (Ed.). (2012). Current knowledge and best practices for telepractice. *The Volta Review, 112*(2), 191–442.

Swanepoel, D. W., & Hall, J. W. (2010). A systematic review of telehealth applications in audiology. *Telemedicine and e-Health, 16*(2), 181–200.

Theodoros, D. (2013). Speech-language pathology and telerehabilitation. In S. Kumar & E. R. Cohn (Eds.), *Telerehabilitation* (pp. 311–323). London, UK: Springer.

Towey, M. (2013). Speech therapy telepractice. In S. Kumar & E. R. Cohn (Eds.), *Telerehabilitation* (pp. 101–123). London, UK: Springer.

Tye-Murray, N. (2009). *Foundations of aural rehabilitation: Children, adults, and their family members* (3rd ed.). New York, NY: Delmar Cengage Learning.

Tye-Murray, N. (2015). *Foundations of aural rehabilitation: Children, adults, and their family members* (4th ed.). New York, NY: Delmar Cengage Learning.

Yoshinaga-Itano, C., & Gravel, J. S. (2001). The evidence for universal hearing screening. *American Journal of Audiology, 10*(2), 62–63.

Yoshinaga-Itano, C., Sedey, A. L., Coutler, D. K., & Mehl, A. L. (1998). Language of early-and later-identified children with hearing loss. *Pediatrics, 102*, 1161–1171.

Wade, V., & Eliott, J. (2012). The role of the champion in telehealth service development: A qualitative analysis. *Journal of Telemedicine and Telecare, 18*, 490–492.

Waite, M., Cahill, L. M., Theodoros, D. G., Busuttin, S., & Russell, T. G. (2006). A pilot study of online assessment of childhood speech disorders. *Journal of Telemedicine and Telecare, 12*(Suppl. 3), 92–94.

Waite, M., Theodoros, D., Russell, T., & Cahill, L. (2010). Internet-based telehealth assessment of language using the CELF-4. *Language, Speech, and Hearing Services in Schools, 41*, 445–458.

Weiss, D., Tilin, F. J., & Morgan, M. J. (2014). *The interprofessional health care team: Leadership and development*. Burlington, MA: Jones & Bartlett Learning.

Winters, J. M., & Winters, J. M. (2004). A telehomecare model for optimizing rehabilitation outcomes. *Telemedicine Journal and e-Health, 10*(2), 200–212.

8

Potential for Telepractice in Audiology: A Review of Applications in Early Hearing Detection and Intervention Programs

Emma Rushbrooke and Beth Atkinson

Key Points

- Telepractice has many applications in the area of teleaudiology.
- Research and case examples from the literature demonstrate both the efficacy and effectiveness of teleaudiology in the area of early hearing detection and intervention (EHDI).
- EHDI programs can reduced the average age of confirmation of hearing loss from 24 months to 3 months (Punch, n.d.; Tharpe, 2013) with the aim of fitting hearing technology and enrollment in an early intervention program by 6 months of age.
- Early detection and intervention impacts positively on outcomes for children born with hearing loss.
- Limited access to hearing health care specialists will impact negatively on outcomes for children born with

hearing loss, and telepractice may offer the solution to bridge the gap.
- Telepractice has the potential to improve continuity of care in the delivery of EHDI services.
- Telepractice can assist in reducing the number of infants lost to follow-up after newborn hearing screening.

Telepractice in hearing health care is gaining acceptance around the world. Although it is generally acknowledged that more research in this area of specialization is required (Swanepoel & Hall, 2010), the changes in technology, improved connectivity, and the computerization of diagnostic audiology equipment have resulted in more teleaudiology applications. And, by extension, more peer-reviewed research publications are emerging (Krumm & Syms, 2011; Ribera & Krumm, 2002). When reviewing this research, it is important to consider not only the efficacy of this approach but also the effectiveness. Although these terms are often used interchangeably, Singal, Higgins, and Waljee (2014) state that research studies can be placed on a continuum, progressing from efficacy trials to effectiveness trials. "Efficacy can be defined as the performance of an intervention under ideal and controlled circumstances, whereas effectiveness refers to its performance under 'real-world' conditions" (p. 1). It is important to understand that efficacy and effectiveness are not isolated but instead overlap, and both need to be considered when assessing a telepractice model of service delivery (Fryback & Thornbury, 1991).

The capacity to deliver hearing health care services to all those in need is limited by the number of qualified audiologists, geography, and lifestyle barriers of the patients (Goulious & Patuzzi, 2008; Swanepoel et al., 2010). Teleaudiology has the potential to extend the service provider's reach with quality services comparable to those delivered face-to-face (i.e., in person). The field of teleaudiology has many applications, including newborn hearing screening, diagnostic and screening assessments, teleotoscopy, hearing technology fittings, rehabilitation, counseling, technology troubleshooting, balance assessments, tinnitus management, education and prevention, and data management and administration. A systematic review of telehealth applications in audiology performed by Swanepoel and Hall (2010) showed that hearing screening, diagnosis, and intervention were feasible and reliable across different ages and patient populations. This chapter examines some of the current applications of teleaudiology in the area of early hearing detection and intervention (EHDI) and considers both the efficacy and effectiveness of these applications. In addition, the beneficial change that a telepractice approach can facilitate in meeting the urgent needs of infants born with hearing loss and their families is highlighted. Although this overview specifically relates to EHDI, much of the discussion can be transferred or is applicable to other applications in the area of teleaudiology.

Why Early Hearing Detection and Intervention (EHDI)?

As information and communication technology continue to progress and evolve, evidence is emerging that teleaudiology applications can meet the full range of diagnostic hearing assessments required for infants born with hearing loss (Swanepeol & Hall, 2010; Swanepoel et al., 2010). However, before we look at these applications, it is important to understand the need for EHDI and the urgency of accessible and timely services. Hearing loss occurs at a rate of 1 to 2 in every 1,000 births in developed countries and in developing countries at a rate of 5 to 6 per 1,000 newborns (Mehl & Thomson, 1998; Patel & Feldman, 2014; World Health Organization [WHO], 2010). Congenital hearing loss is the most common detectable disability in newborns. Congenital hearing loss is 20 times more common in newborns than the metabolic blood disorder phenylketonuria (PKU) and 15 times more common than sickle cell anemia. Both PKU and sickle cell anemia are disorders for which screening is routinely performed (Minnesota Health Department, 2014; Patel & Feldman, 2014). However, although some developed countries, such as Australia and the United States, have established EHDI programs (National Institutes of Health, 2013; Punch, n.d.), this is not the case in many parts of the world (Swanepoel et al., 2010).

What Are the Benefits of Early Hearing Detection and Intervention?

Early detection and intervention for infants born with hearing loss is essential to enable them to reach their full developmental potential. Without early access to sound and specialized intervention, children born with hearing loss demonstrate devastating and irreversible deficits in listening and spoken language, cognition, literacy, and social skills (Downs & Yoshinaga-Itano, 1999; Mehl & Thomson, 1998; Patel & Feldman, 2014). Before the introduction of newborn hearing screening in countries like Australia, the average age of hearing loss confirmation was 24 months, and postintroduction is now 3 months (Punch, n.d.; Tharpe, 2013). In the 21st century, we are seeing that innovation is leading to even greater opportunities in the early diagnosis and treatment of congenital hearing loss, allowing these children to achieve their full potential developmentally, communicatively, and academically.

The evidence suggests that more than 90% of children born with hearing loss have the physical ear structures that enable them to benefit from the use of modern hearing technology (Adunka et al., 2006; Rance, 2005). There is also an ever-expanding range of hearing technology available. This means that, regardless of the degree or type of hearing loss, more than ever before, hearing health professionals can meet the specific needs of the majority of children with hearing loss.

Neuroscience research has found that the auditory brain starts developing in utero and is "prewired" to accept and process sound. The brain connections that allow a child to understand speech are formed and shaped by auditory experience. If stimulated through meaningful sound, the auditory brain develops multiple neural pathways permanently (Dornan, 2015; Dornan, Hickson, Murdoch, & Houston, 2009). Patel and Feldman (2014) note that the evidence shows that auditory deprivation in early infancy results in structural and functional reorganization at a cortical level (Dornan, 2015; Dornan et al., 2009; Gordon, Jiwani, & Papsin, 2013; Sininger, Doyle, & Moore, 1999). Auditory brain development in babies is very rapid, and optimal developmental periods need to be considered. Because of this factor, together with optimized auditory stimulation and intervention, a child's ability to hear, learn to listen, understand, and develop spoken language can be achieved. Optimal developmental periods are limited windows of time, which usually close early in a child's life. Within these periods, massive interconnecting of neural pathways and pruning of unwanted or unused neural connections occur. The optimal period for the development of listening and spoken language is from birth to 3.5 years (Sharma, Dorman, & Kral, 2005; Sharma, Dorman, & Spahr, 2002). The Joint Committee on Infant Hearing (JCIH) recommends screening all newborns before 1 month of age, performing a diagnostic evaluation on those who fail screening and prescribing appropriate hearing technology before 3 months, and initiating intervention services for infants with permanent hearing loss before 6 months (JCIH, 2007). In view of this, equity of access to hearing health care professionals is essential to meet these recommended targets and to enable early access to intervention for children born with hearing loss. Telepractice has the potential to offer a solution, not only in the delivery of screening and diagnostic hearing services but to also assist with the delivery of early intervention services.

Advances in diagnosis and hearing technology allow us to take advantage of normal developmental processes by stimulating the auditory or hearing part of the brain in a timely and dedicated manner. The majority of children who have access to early identification and targeted and specialized listening and spoken language intervention will develop spoken language outcomes on par with their normally hearing peers (Dornan et al., 2009; Dornan, 2015). However, all of this knowledge and innovation is worthless if the child and family do not have access to appropriate and timely audiological, medical, and early intervention services. Sadly, this is the case in many parts of the world, which leads to undetected and untreated hearing loss having devastating effects on young children and their families. Limited access to services impacts across the life span, from a global perspective; approximately 80% of people with hearing loss cannot access hearing health care services, because they live in developing countries where audiologists or other hearing health care workers are not available (Fagan & Jacobs, 2009; Goulios & Patuzzi, 2008; Swanepoel, 2013; Swanepoel, Hall, & Biagio, 2011). In addition, although newborn hearing screening has become the standard of care in many parts of the world, some programs report that almost half of the babies who do not pass their newborn hearing screen are lost to follow-up after their initial screen (Houston, Behl, & Walters, 2013), thus negating the advantage of early diagnosis. Improving access and making follow-up easier will go some way to assist in reducing the number of newborns lost to follow-up.

EHDI Program Diagnostic Assessments

As noted, EHDI programs have been established in many countries around the world to screen and diagnose infants with hearing loss. There are two types of audiological tests that are generally recognized as the standard of care for newborn hearing screening in infants. These are otoacoustic emissions (OAEs) and automated auditory brainstem response testing (AABR) (Krumm, Huffman, Dick, & Klich, 2008). The WHO (2010) has stated that universal newborn hearing screening using OAE or AABR should be the goal for all countries. As these assessments are automated and objective, they do not require a response from the infant. These objective measures make them ideal for infant hearing screening. In addition, the results of the screening test do not require interpretation as the automated equipment provides a pass or refer (fail) result. As such, this testing method is suitable for nonspecialists to administer, that is, trained screeners or screening assistants who are not audiologists. This is the model that is used in many programs, increasing both flexibility and accessibility. However, the success of these programs relies on the availability of trained staff to perform the screening tests. In contrast, some rural and remote hospitals may be so limited by the staff they have available that newborn hearing screenings cannot be provided (Krumm et al., 2008; Ramkumar, Hall, Nagarajan, Shankarnarayan, & Kumaravelu, 2013; Winston & Ditty, 2014). In areas where infant screening is not available, many new parents may not be willing or may find it difficult to travel to testing sites. In cases such as this, an alternative telepractice approach is an option that should be considered (Krumm et al., 2008).

As previously noted, it is essential that families have timely follow-up to diagnostic hearing assessment if their babies do not pass newborn hearing screening; a child referred for further testing can have as great as a 1 in 12 chance of having a hearing loss (Houston et al., 2013; UCDavis Teleaudiology Program, 2012). In addition, the parents or caregivers may experience increased levels of anxiety or stress until diagnostic tests are performed, highlighting the importance of effective counseling and rapid follow-up. Timely access can be a challenge for families living in regional and remote areas, where a dearth of pediatric hearing specialists and geography create obstacles or barriers (Kennedy, 2011; UCDavis Teleaudiology Program, 2012).

Follow-up diagnostic confirmation testing uses a number of electrophysiological assessments such as auditory brainstem response (ABR) testing. As these assessments use computer-based systems, they are ideal for telepractice using remote access software but must be performed or supervised by a pediatric audiologist. Krishnan (2009) notes that one of the major challenges to successful implementation of EHDI programs is the shortage of specialist pediatric audiologists.

Evidence in the Literature to Support a Telepractice Model of Delivery

The screening and diagnostic applications of teleaudiology now cover the entire test battery, enabling a possible solution to the dilemma of unequal access. Evidence is emerging to demonstrate the efficacy and effectiveness of a teleaudiology application to this area of service delivery. Examples of the provision of these diagnostic assessments (through telepractice) in the literature demonstrate the feasibility of a teleaudiology model of delivery. Elangovan (2005) examined the real-time assessment of OAEs. The recordings were under two conditions for each individual ear (i.e., with the conventional system and the tele-OAE system). Both tests were performed by audiologists, and the order of testing was counterbalanced among test ears (Elangovan, 2005). Participants had no knowledge of which system was being used in the assessment procedure as the audiologist on site with the patient placed the testing probe in the patient's ear for both the remote and face-to-face procedure. The results showed good reliability for both systems; the audiometric results obtained in local and remote conditions were not statistically different (Elangovan, 2005). The author did, however, note that trained audiologists performed the role of the facilitator at the test site, and as such, evaluation under "real-world" conditions is needed to demonstrate the effectiveness of this mode of service delivery.

Towers, Pisa, Froelich, and Krumm (2005) examined the reliability of ABR testing via the Internet by comparing results obtained locally in the conventional manner with those from a remote site. Statistical analysis of the data obtained in the trials showed a strong correlation between data collected at both sites, which again showed the potential for this technology to obtain accurate results at a distance. Although these studies show the efficacy and feasibility of using this method, again validation using trained on-site facilitators who are not audiologists needs further investigation as this would be the model of delivery to an area that does not have access to a local audiologist.

In a study conducted by Krumm et al. (2008), hearing screening services were delivered using both a traditional face-to-face model and a real-time (synchronous) teleaudiology approach in a group on infants. The study used hearing screening assessments that are typically performed in newborn hearing screening programs. The assessments used were distortion product otoacoustic emissions (DPOAEs) and AABR. The group of infants had the screening assessments performed twice, both face-to-face and using a teleaudiology method to enable comparison of outcome. An audiologist was available to perform the assessments on the newborns in the face-to-face condition at a regional medical center. Another audiologist provided the same assessments through remote computing from Utah State University, which was approximately 200 km from the subjects. The audiologist who was present with the newborn in the face-to-face condition applied the AABR recording electrodes and inserted the earphones and the DPOAE probe tip. All of these equipment applications were used for both the face-to-face and remote testing conditions. The software determined whether a "pass" or "refer" was achieved based on computerized algorithms, and results indicated identical screening results for all infants ($n = 30$, aged 11–45 days) when face-to-face and remote test conditions were compared. This study identified some limitations, including the use of an audiologist for the telepractice condition at the patient site. As previously noted, typically a trained assistant would be utilized for this role. Overall, this study supports the use of teleaudiology for conducting remote hearing screening in infants.

Ramkumar et al. (2013) demonstrated the feasibility of using a mobile van, with satellite connectivity, to perform real-time remote diagnostic ABRs. Trained health care workers assisted and the ABR equipment was controlled by an audiologist at a hospital site. Twenty four newborns were tested and recordings made via telepractice were compared to those obtained face-to-face. Results showed no significant difference between the recordings. Videoconferencing was used to observe the testing of the newborn, including skin preparation for recording electrodes and electrode placement. The testing procedure and the baby's movements could be observed while testing was taking place in real time. Although the study showed the effectiveness of this approach, by using trained facilitators at the patient/client location, a limitation of the study included that fact that testing was performed over a short distance only, that is, only 1 km (0.62 miles) from the hospital with a reliable power supply, and as such, further investigation of the effectiveness of the service from more remote sites is required. However, despite these limitations, the study demonstrated a flexible model to improve access in rural and remote sites (Ramkumar et al., 2013).

In 2009, Glenrose Rehabilitation Hospital (GRH) Audiology Department reported a collaboration with Alberta Health Services Clinical Telehealth and Northern Lights Regional Health Centre (NLRHC) at Fort McMurray to offer diagnostic ABR testing using telepractice to improve access to this hospital-based service in a remote community. Using secure videoconferencing and remote desktop access, GRH audiologists performed remote diagnostic ABR tests in real time. The hospital reported that the remote ABR service delivery model had a significant positive impact on the families offered this service, in relation to improving accessibility to tertiary-level services in their community and considerable cost savings, related to travel (Kennedy, 2011). It was also reported that because the program reduced the need for families to travel long and often uncomfortable distances with a newborn, testing outcomes were obtained more efficiently and the number of appointments required was often reduced. Infants need to be asleep for ABR testing, and as such, families are required to keep their baby awake until they arrive at the testing center. This is particularly difficult, and traveling long distances can result in appointments being rebooked, due to an inability to settle the infant into a sleeping state (Kennedy, 2011). Multiple appointments to complete tests can place considerable strain on parents and the family unit both emotionally and financially. Houston, Behl, and Walters (2013) noted that a survey conducted with state EHDI coordinators by the National Center for Hearing Assessment and Management (NCHAM) showed that 42% had some type of telehealth efforts either under way or planned. They reported that the use of audiology telepractice to conduct diagnostic ABRs remotely was the second most common service implemented or in the planning stages (after teleintervention). In order to ensure timely delivery of services from properly trained professionals, EHDI coordinators noted that there were ongoing plans to either expand or implement remote hearing aid programming and/or mapping of implantable hearing technology through models of audiology telepractice (Houston et al., 2013). This planned expansion of services highlights the fact that all services related to EHDI can potentially be delivered via telepractice. In addition to improved access and more timely follow-up diagnostic assessment, telepractice models offer other advantages, such as training and support of EHDI professionals and the ability to provide a second opinion for difficult diagnostic cases to sole or isolated audiologists (Sutton & Wood, 2011; Campbell & Sawyer, 2009). (Editors' note: Discussions about remote hearing aid fittings, cochlear implant programming, professional training, and mentoring are covered in other chapters in this book.)

An effective teleaudiology program can also further promote greater continuity of services and care. Medical and health information relating to the infant and family can be shared securely via telepractice (Krumm, Ribera, & Schmiedge, 2005). This allows the hearing health care professional access to relevant case history information and the ability to communicate with other professionals involved in the provision of care. Behl, Tharpe, Hayes, and Hunting (2013) note that consistent communication with the audiologist and other related professionals is very important to families.

In response to the potential benefits of telepractice, ASHA developed a position paper that supports the use of telepractice by audiologists (ASHA, 2005a, 2005b).

Early Intervention: Re/Habilitation

Diagnosis and hearing technology alone is not enough it to maximize the developmental outcome of a child born with hearing loss; they must be coupled with targeted and specialized early intervention. More than 90% of children with hearing loss are born to normally hearing parents (Mitchell & Karchmer, 2004), and for most of these families, they will choose a listening and spoken language (LSL) intervention option. If parents desire an LSL outcome for their child with hearing loss, an educational approach that emphasizes the development of auditory brain pathways through listening and spoken language is necessary (Cole & Flexer, 2007).

Like audiology, access to listening and spoken language specialists (LSLSs) is also difficult, and families of infants and children with hearing loss are often challenged to find qualified specialists in this field. Houston and Perigoe (2010) note that there is a shortage of professionals with appropriate knowledge and skills to deliver evidence-based early intervention services to this population. These re/habilitation services can also be delivered through telepractice, and many services are employing this approach. (Editors' note: This model of service delivery is discussed further in Chapter 7 of this book.)

Summary

A review of some of the research in the area of EHDI shows that the diagnostic hearing assessments and other related interventions lend themselves well to a telepractice model of service delivery. Improved access is likely to lead to quicker follow-up, a reduced age of diagnosis, and more timely initiation of appropriate early intervention.

Although much of the literature reviewed demonstrated validity and efficacy, one of the limitations noted was that further peer-reviewed and published research was needed to show outcomes using trained assistants rather than audiologists at the local sites, which would demonstrate both the efficacy and effectiveness of this "real-world" model.

Overall, the application of telepractice to the area of EHDI has the potential to not only improve access but to also reduce the number of families lost to follow-up, increase continuity of care, and reduce parental stress in some cases.

References

Adunka, O., Roush, P., Teagle, H., Brown, C., Zdanski, C., & Jewells, V. (2006). Internal auditory canal morphology in children with cochlear nerve deficiency. *Otology & Neurotology, 27*(6), 793–801.

American Speech-Language-Hearing Association. (2005a). *Audiologists providing clinical services via telepractice* [Position statement]. Retrieved from http://www.asha.org/policy

American Speech-Language-Hearing Association. (2005b). *Audiologists providing clinical services via telepractice* [Technical report]. Retrieved from http://www.asha.org/policy

Behl, D., Tharpe, A.-M., Hayes, D., & Hunting, V. (2013, April). *The role of teleaudiology in supporting access to care.* PowerPoint presentation, EHDI Meeting, Glendale, AZ.

Campbell, P. H., & Sawyer, L. B. (2009). Changing early intervention providers' home visiting skills through participation in professional development. *Topics in Early Childhood Special Education, 28*(4), 219–234. doi:10.1177/0271121408328481

Cole, E., & Flexer, C. (2007). *Children with hearing loss: Developing listening and talking, birth to six.* San Diego, CA: Plural.

Dornan, D. (2015). Current considerations on neural development and hearing loss in young children. *ENT & Audiology News, 23*(6), 75–78.

Dornan, D., Hickson, L., Murdoch, B., & Houston, T. (2009). Longitudinal study of speech and language for children with hearing loss in auditory-verbal therapy programs. *The Volta Review, 109*, 61–85.

Downs, M. P., & Yoshinaga-Itano, C. (1999). The efficacy of early identification and intervention for children with hearing impairment. *Pediatric Clinics of North America, 46*(1), 79–87.

Elangovan, S. (2005). Telehearing and the Internet. *Seminars in Hearing, 26*, 19–25.

Fagan, J. J., & Jacobs, M. (2009). Survey of ENT services in Africa: need for a comprehensive intervention. *Global Health Action, 2*. doi:10.3402/gha.v2i0.1932. Retrieved from http://www.ncbi.nlm.nih .gov/pmc/articles/PMC2779942/

Fryback, D. G., & Thornbury, J. R. (1991). The efficacy of diagnostic imaging. *Medical Decision Making, 11*, 88.

Gordon, K. A., Jiwani, S., & Papsin, B. C. (2013). Benefits and detriments of unilateral cochlear implant use on bilateral auditory development in children who are deaf. *Frontiers in Psychology, 4*, article 719.

Goulios, H., & Patuzzi, R. B. (2008). Audiology education and practice from an international perspective. *International Journal of Audiology, 47*, 647–664.

Houston, K. T., Behl, D., & Walters, K. Z. (2013). Using telepractice to improve outcomes for children with hearing loss & their families. In L. R. Schmeltz (Ed.), *NCHAM@Book: A resource guide for Early Hearing Detection and Intervention (EHDI)*. Retrieved December 3, 2014, from http://www.infanthearing.org/ehdi-ebook/2013_ebook/ 18Chapter17UsingTelepractive2013.pdf

Houston, K. T., & Perigoe, C. (2010). Future directions in professional preparation and development. *The Volta Review, 110*(2), 339–340.

Joint Committee on Infant Hearing (JCIH). (2007). Year 2007 position statement: Principles and guidelines for early hearing detection and intervention programs. *Pediatrics, 120*(4), 898–921.

Kennedy, G. (2011). Two-city teamwork brings high-tech hearing test to infants. Alberta Health Services. *News and Events*. Retrieved January 2015 from http://www.albertahealthservices.ca/4658.asp

Krishnan, L. A. (2009). Universal newborn hearing screening follow-up: A university clinic perspective. *American Journal of Audiology, 18*, 89–98.

Krumm, M., Huffman, T., Dick, K., & Klich, R. (2008).Telemedicine for audiology screening of infants. *Journal of Telemedicine and Telecare, 14*(2), 102–104.

Krumm, M., Ribera, J., & Schmiedge, J. (2005). Using a telehealth medium for objective hearing testing: Implications for supporting rural universal newborn hearing screening programs. *Seminars in Hearing, 26*, 3–12.

Krumm, M., & Syms, M. (2011). Teleaudiology. *Otolaryngology Clinics of North America, 44*(6), 1297–1304.

Mehl, A. L., & Thomson, V. (1998). Newborn hearing screening: The great omission. *Pediatrics, 101*(1), E4.

Minnesota Department of Health. (2014). *Hearing screening online training program: Newborn hearing screening.* Retrieved December 3, 2014, from http://www.health.state.mn.us/divs/fh/mch/web course/hearing/newborn1.cfm

Mitchell, R. E., & Karchmer, M. A. (2004). Chasing the mythical ten percent: Parental hearing status of deaf and hard of hearing students in the United States. *Sign Language Studies, 4*(2), 138–163.

National Institutes of Health (NIH). (2013). *NIH fact sheet: Newborn hearing screening.* Retrieved December 2014 from http://report.nih .gov/NIHfactsheets/ViewFactSheet.aspx?csid=104

Patel, H., & Feldman, M. (2014). Universal newborn hearing screening. *Paediatrics and Child Health, 16*(5), 301–305.

Punch, R. (n.d.). *Universal newborn hearing screening. Victorian Deaf Education Unit.* Retrieved December 2014 from http://www.deaf education.vic.edu.au/Documents/Resources/UniNBHearScreen.pdf

Ramkumar, V., Hall, J. W., Nagarajan, R., Shankarnarayan, V. C., & Kuma-ravelu, S. (2013). Tele-ABR using a satellite connection in a mobile van for newborn hearing testing. *Journal of Telemedicine and Telecare, 19*(5), 233–237.

Rance, G. (2005). Auditory neuropathy/dys-synchrony and its perceptual consequences. *Trends in Amplification, 9,* 1–43.

Ribera, J., & Krumm, M. (2002). Telepractice in audiology. *Audiology Online.* Retrieved January 4, 2015, from http://www.audiologyon line.com/articles/telepractice-in-audiology-1184

Sharma, A., Dorman, M. F., & Kral, A. (2005). The influence of a sensitive period on central auditory development in children with unilateral and bilateral cochlear implants. *Hearing Research, 203,* 134–143.

Sharma, A., Dorman, M. F., & Spahr, A. J. (2002). A sensitive period for the development of the central auditory system in children with cochlear implants: Implications for age of implantation. *Ear and Hearing, 23*(6), 532–539.

Singal, A. G., Higgins, P. D. R., & Waljee, A. K. (2014). A primer on effectiveness and efficacy trials. *Clinical and Translational Gastro-enterology, 5,* e45.

Sininger, Y. S., Doyle, K. J., & Moore, J. K. (1999). The case for early identification of hearing loss in children: Auditory system development, experimental auditory deprivation, and development of speech perception and hearing. *Pediatric Clinics of North America, 46,* 1–14.

Sutton, G., & Wood, S. (2011). *Improving the quality of newborn ABRs. Report on NHSP ABR quality improvement pilots in East of England & Greater Manchester 2009–11.* Retrieved May 11, 2014, from http:// hearing.screening.nhs.uk

Swanepoel, D. (2013). 20Q: Audiology to the people—combining technology and connectivity for services by telehealth. *AudiologyOnline,* Article 12183. Retrieved February 2, 2014, from http://www.audiol ogyonline.com

Swanepoel, D., Clark, J., Koekemoer, D., Hall, J., Krumm, M., Ferrari, D., . . . Barajas, J. J. (2010). Telehealth in audiology: The need and potential to reach underserved communities. *International Journal of Audiology, 49,* 195–202.

Swanepoel, D., & Hall, J. (2010). A systematic review of telehealth applications in audiology. *Telemedicine Journal and e-Health, 16,* 181–200.

Swanepoel, D., Hall, J., & Biagio, L. (2011). Tele-audiology offers great promise in reaching underserved people globally. *Hearing Views @ Hearing Health Matters.* Retrieved April 8, 2014, from http:// hearinghealthmatters.org/hearingviews/2011/tele-audiology-offers-great-promise

Tharpe, A.-M. (2013, December). *A quick look back and a charge going forward.* PowerPoint slide presentation, Vanderbilt University School of Medicine. Retrieved January 2015 from http://www.slideshare .net/Phonak/a-quick-look-back-and-a-charge-going-forward1

Towers, A. D., Pisa, J., Froelich, T. M., & Krumm, M. (2005). The reliability of click-evoked and frequency-specific auditory brainstem response testing using telehealth technology. *Seminars in Hearing, 26*(1), 26–34.

UC Davis Teleaudiology Program. (2012). *The California Tele-Audiology Program.* Retrieved December 2014 from http://citris-uc.org/the-california-tele-audiology-program/

Winston, R., & Ditty, K. M. (2014). Newborn hearing screening. In L. R. Schmeltz (Ed.), *NCHAM@Book: A resource guide for Early Hearing Detection and Intervention (EHDI).* Retrieved December 3, 2014, from http://www.infanthearing.org/ehdi-ebook/2014_ebook/2-Chapter2NewbornHearing2014.pdf

World Health Organization. (2010). *Newborn and infant hearing screening: Current issues and guiding principles for action.* Retrieved December 3, 2014, from http://www.who.int/blindness/publica tions/Newborn_and_Infant_Hearing_Screening_Report

9

Maximizing Professional Development Opportunities Using Telepractice

Jackie Brown and Carolyn Evans

Key Points

- Increased Internet connectivity and improvements in telecommunication technology in the 21st century are providing greater opportunities for professional training and development, regardless of location.
- Professionals need ongoing professional training to be available in a variety of delivery modes.
- Professionals need access to peer-to-peer support as well as supervision and mentoring.
- Telepractice has the potential to overcome difficulties with availability and flexibility of access for professionals seeking training, supervision, and mentoring.
- The use of a range of telepractice techniques and strategies ensures the accommodation of different learning styles.

Terminology

There are a number of ways of defining telepractice terms. In this chapter, eTraining refers to the delivery of training and educational programs, via the Internet, to improve the knowledge and skills of qualified professionals in order to better equip them to meet their role requirements. eSupervision refers to the formalized supervision provided by a senior practitioner, via the Internet, to an undergraduate or intern, overseeing their service provision to clients. eMentoring refers to the support provided by a senior practitioner, via the Internet, to a qualified professional who requires observation, guidance, and feedback in order to further develop skills in a specialized area of practice.

A blended cyber model uses both asynchronous and synchronous techniques. Asynchronous techniques refers to learning tasks, such as readings, assignments, and examinations being loaded electronically for the students to access in their own time, as long as the final time frames are met. There is no personal interaction between the various parties. A synchronous model, however, allows all parties to interact with each other, such as via online chat rooms or webinars. This communication may be through speaking or through instant messaging (Hrastinski, 2008).

Webinar refers to a presentation, lecture, or seminar that is transmitted over the Internet and allows for interaction to occur in real time between the presenter and attendees. A webcast, on the other hand, is prerecorded material with little or no ability for the participants to be interactive (Romero, 2010; South Carolina CPA, 2014).

Introduction

The World Health Organization (WHO) estimates that there are 360 million people worldwide with a significant hearing loss, representing 5.3% of the world's population (WHO, 2013a, 2013b). When member states were surveyed, the paucity of hearing health care professionals was evident, with 29% of respondents having one or fewer ear, nose, and throat (ENT) specialists per million people and 51% having one or fewer audiologists per million. The availability of training facilities for audiologists was reported as 41% overall, ranging from 14% in low-income areas to 70% in high-income areas. Even with the 1995 WHO resolution to address hearing health care, in particular preventable hearing loss, by 2013, only 40% of member states reported the presence of national policies or programs focusing on hearing health (WHO, 1995). Lack of financial or human resources and other health priorities were most often cited as the reason behind the lack of initiative in this area; however, absence of need was never highlighted. This is echoed in a worldwide survey conducted by Goulios and Patuzzi (2008), who found that audiological support was reported as insufficient in 86% of countries. The two main contributing factors identified in their study were a lack of funding and a priority toward other health initiatives. Unavailability of clinical training placements was also highlighted as a reason for the shortage of audiological services. Even in the United States, availability of clinical placements has been highlighted as one of the major obstacles to increasing the numbers of experienced practicing clinicians within Doctor of Audiology (AuD) programs (Windmill, 2013). Clinical placements allow for theoretical knowledge to be translated into practice and for skilled clinicians to impart expertise in less taught skills, such as interacting with clients and other health professionals.

The development of accessible, cost-effective educational programs is essential to train quality staff to implement, run, and grow health care initiatives. The evolution of connectivity to the Internet has created a portal by which this may be possible. According to World Internet Usage and Population statistics ("Internet World Stats," 2012), Internet usage has grown over 500% worldwide, with over 3,000% growth in Africa alone for the period from 2000 to 2012. Additionally, the total number of subscribers to mobile broadband worldwide has risen from 2.3 billion in 2008 to 3.4 billion in 2013, with predictions that there will be over 3.9 billion by 2017 (Page, Molina, & Jones, 2013). In terms of professional development, this means access: access to training courses, access to journal articles, access to recorded lectures, access to instructional videos, access to peer support, and access without travel and without high cost.

The following is a discussion of the options available for online learning in terms of continuing education and professional development in the field of audiology. Examples from Hear and Say are provided to demonstrate the potential afforded by online delivery of training, supervision, and mentoring.

Professional Development: Opportunities and Challenges

Continuing professional development is important to ensure prolonged currency of knowledge, skills, and competencies in one's profession. It is an ongoing process and is an obligation that continues throughout a professional's career. In the field of audiology, ongoing professional development to maintain certification and licensure is mandated by professional organizations; however, it is also the personal responsibility of professionals and will assist them to deliver quality services that should result in high levels of client and clinician satisfaction. Professional development through education is a source of empowerment; however, access to high-quality opportunities can be challenging for audiologists, as many will be restricted by distance, expense, and time. In response to these challenges, professional development opportunities through telepractice offer an alternative avenue of access.

As a case example, in order to practice as an audiologist in Australia, with full access to funding bodies, membership in Audiology Australia must be gained and a Certificate of Clinical Practice (CCP) approved and maintained. Applicants (Master of Audiology graduates) must complete a clinical internship program, whereby supervised clinical skills are documented over a 48-week period and competencies graded. Once the CCP has been obtained, an audiologist must submit Continuing Professional Development (CPD) points biennially to maintain eligibility for Audiology Australia membership. CPD points may be obtained, for example, from attending a conference, lecture, or product training; clinical supervision or teaching; or mentoring or participating in research. (See http://www.audiology.asn .au for a full list of possible activities with CPD point values, retrieved April 27, 2014.)

The easiest way to obtain CPD points is to attend the Audiology Australia conference, where a maximum of 40 points may be obtained toward the required 50 points; however, the costs involved in attendance are prohibitive for many audiologists. Table 9–1 shows 2014 fees for the Audiology Australia conference and corresponding audiology society conferences worldwide. If the conference venue is not local, there are also the additional expenses of travel, accommodation, and dining in addition to the loss of income the audiology service provider would incur for study leave and from reduction in client fees.

With the advent of teleconferencing technology, access to lectures presented at conferences is improving. The 2013 British Academy of Audiology (BAA) conference, for example, had a total of 73 presentations, of which 12 were recorded and made available to access online with another 45 available to view as PowerPoint presentations. This availability eliminates the costs of travel and conference fees, leaving only the challenge of time and accessibility to contend with. Relevance of material is important and must be taken into consideration when considering the

Table 9–1. Examples of Conference Fees in 2014 for Audiological Societies

Society	Location	Conference Fee in USD	Conference Fee in AUD
SAC (Speech-Language and Audiology Canada)	Ottawa, ON, Canada	$607	$651
ASHA (American Speech and Hearing Association)	Orlando, FL, USA	$860	$922
Audiology Australia	Brisbane, Australia	$1,000	$1,072
BAA (British Academy of Audiology)	Bournemouth, UK	$588	$635

costs involved in attendance. Diversity in the skills and needs of audiological health care professionals and hearing health priorities means a "one-size-fits-all" approach to education is impossible. Goulios and Patuzzi (2008), in a survey of audiology services, found that the education level of practitioners could be divided into four subsets: (1) medically qualified practitioners specialized in the field of ENT or audiology, (2) university-qualified practitioners with a degree in audiology, (3) graduates from a technical or vocational college or school, and (4) practitioners with a nonmedical degree but with some health care practice as part of their job role. This diversity stems from the emphasis placed on the audiologist in hearing health service delivery relative to other professionals. For example, the ENT specialist may be responsible for the majority of audiological service provision in some countries (Goulios & Patuzzi, 2008). Rather than attending a conference where only a portion of the content may be relevant to a given professional, it is now possible to access webinars and webcasts on a myriad of topics. Webinars involve synchronous delivery of training material and the option for online attendees to interact with an expert speaker. Webcasts allow access as required but no real-time interaction. Countless platforms support both modes of delivery, such as AudiologyOnline (http://www.audiologyonline.com), Cochlear HOPE (http://hope.cochlearamericas.com), and VIP e-Learning on the Phonak website (http://www.phonakpro.com), The Hearing Education and Research Network or HEARnet (http://www.hearingcrc.org/communication/hearnet), created by the HEARing CRC to provide information about HEARing CRC research outcomes, may be accessed free of charge. Although audiological societies are generally accepting of online content as contributing to continuing education point collection, there are stipulations for its inclusion. Topics must be relevant to audiology or involve fields that impact clinical practice. For example, a clinician working in a pediatric cochlear implant program may benefit from lectures by a psychologist or social worker aiming to enhance discussions with families during candidacy assessments. Event coordinators may seek prior approval of CPD status, so that clinicians are aware of the point value prior to participation.

Social media sites, such as Facebook, provide an opportunity for professionals or clients, or a combination of both, to interact in online discussion groups that are generally geared toward a particular topic with restricted access. For example, students participating in a training program may be required to join a group to facilitate discussion or follow tutorials. Behl, Houston, and Stredler-Brown (2012) describe the establishment of a learning community to generate support for professionals involved in telepractice for children with hearing loss. Initial contact to establish rapport between professionals and build a "sense of community" involved a face-to-face gathering over a 1.5-day period. Professionals then participated in monthly phone conferences for a 6-month period, following which a Facebook group was set up to facilitate ongoing peer-to-peer support. Facebook is ideal for this purpose as it is easily accessible, with 1.23 billion users worldwide (Hutchinson & Smith, 2014), and allows creation of restricted access groups for text discussion as well as uploading of documents and videos. Applications for hearing health professionals to use social media are vast and undoubtedly underutilized. For example, future directions could include using social media to disseminate regional protocols and outcomes data for programs such as universal newborn hearing screening. Likewise, hearing aid manufacturers could release new product information, software updates, and training schedules. Clinicians could discuss difficult case management scenarios. Perhaps more complex and limiting factors involve the development of specific professional networks with a "sense of community," important for establishing respect and trust of colleagues (Behl et al., 2012), information security, and evaluation of efficacy.

Importance of Peer-to-Peer Support

When faced with referring a patient for audiology services, a general physician looks for the clinic specializing in their client's area of concern: pediatric or adult, assessment or rehabilitation, perhaps as specific as vestibular or auditory processing. In larger towns and cities, there is greater opportunity for clinician specialization due to clinic size and numbers of staff employed. In more remote areas, referrals go to "the" audiologist who is expected to have knowledge covering the entire field of audiology. Utilizing telepractice, through eTraining, eSupervision, and eMentoring, allows the development and expert application of clinical knowledge and skills. Accessing telepractice requires motivation and commitment from both the clinician seeking professional development and the "expert" providing it, but the reduction in costs relating to removal of distance is a strong proponent for success.

eMentoring has an application in verification of auditory brainstem response (ABR) audiometry threshold detection. Although ABR is an objective measure of hearing levels, when determining an ABR threshold, an element of subjectivity is introduced when the clinician makes a judgement as to response presence or absence. High levels of variability between testers have been reported, especially nearing threshold in adverse conditions with high electrical noise or movement artifact (Arnold, 1985; Vidler & Parker, 2004). Given the importance of the results in identifying hearing loss in infants and the subsequent predictions of required gain for hearing aid fitting, it is advantageous to use a peer review process to improve the accuracy of the results. This is generally achieved in an asynchronous manner, whereby traces are printed and marked and then forwarded to another audiologist for review. Sutton and Wood (2011) report on a pilot study carried out as part of the Newborn Hearing Screening Programme (NHSP) in England to test a system of peer review for improving ABR quality. Clinicians were asked to submit ABR traces, which were then reviewed asynchronously for methodology, interpretation, and appropriateness of the recommended follow-up. Just under half of all reviewed traces required further comment from the reviewers, with 3% considered "poor," indicating disagreement with the interpretation and/or management recommended by the clinician, thus highlighting the importance of peer review. Although this pilot was designed as part of a quality assurance program for peer review, it could be adjusted, taking into account the reported limitations, to create an eMentoring program. The authors highlighted limitations for reviewer anonymity, recommending that discussion of results should be encouraged, an important part of any mentoring process. The authors also pointed out the increase in administration time required to create an anonymous record for transfer to an external reviewer. Transfer of records was done via fax and could potentially be simplified using electronic data transfer or upload to a dedicated cloud-based storage system with restricted access such as Dropbox or Google Drive. For clinicians such as new graduates, who require comprehensive guidance, this could be extended to synchronous eMentoring, using videoconferencing software to allow the mentor to observe and have immediate input into the analysis of the waveforms. For clinicians who work in isolation or remotely or who are training in evoked potential assessments but do not have exposure to high volumes of referrals from the screening program, it is crucial to provide ABR waveforms for discussion with an experienced clinician locally, nationally, or internationally.

Peer reviews are not limited to electrophysiology; rather, they can be applied in any area of audiology to ensure current practice is maintained. Clinicians may benefit from discussing difficult cases relating to diagnostic assessments or rehabilitation. New graduates rarely have a full range of clinical competencies at graduation and will benefit from mentoring to help establish expertise. In a survey report determining the use of telepractice among audiologists and speech-language pathologists (American Speech-Language-Hearing Association [ASHA], 2002), nearly 50% of participants indicated that they used telepractice for the purpose of education or training students and 58% for education or training of "other professionals." Undoubtedly, these percentages will have increased since 2002 along with improvements in technology. Synchronous eTraining, eSupervision, and eMentoring are evolving due to accessibility to online videoconferencing systems. Programs such as Skype or Lync allow instant messaging, videoconferencing, voice calls (VoIP), and file sharing, thus facilitating synchronous or asynchronous interaction as long as access to hardware, such as computers, webcams, microphones, and speakers, along with Internet access with reasonable bandwidth, is available.

Counseling plays a significant role in providing an effective audiological service. Whether a clinician is informing families about hearing loss or promoting use of amplification, client satisfaction is increased by competent use of counseling skills. English and Archibold (2014) discuss work from Zolnierek and DiMatteo (2009) in the field of medicine. They found that patients were more likely to adhere to recommendations from medical staff when patient-centered communication strategies were employed. Crandell and Weiner (2002) examined the self-reported improvement in counseling competency following an 8-week distance learning course that examined social, emotional, and psychological concerns both of persons with hearing loss and parents of children with hearing loss. In the final question of the competency scale asking if the class had influenced the clinician's counseling overall, 98.9% of participants indicated some degree of improvement. This is echoed by English and Archibold (2014), who reported a self-determined improvement in audiological counseling skills following participation in a training program that included two 5-hour workshops and 6 weeks of guided independent study. These improvements were also noted 6 months following the completion of the course, indicating meaningful change was initiated by the training. These studies highlight not only the importance of counseling in audiological practice but the ease by which these skills can be obtained and implemented. In an eTraining paradigm, the simulated patient could be presented via videoconferencing software to allow clinicians to develop counseling skills remotely. In a study by Naeve-Velguth, Christensen, and Woods (2013), audiology students participated in a simulated appointment where they were required to give parents (played by an actor) news of an infant's hearing loss. The students found the experience to have a positive impact on identifying counseling strengths and weaknesses, and they were likely to recommend the use of simulated patients to other students. By using this study design, training of the actors could occur within university programs, and clinicians seeking support to strengthen their counseling skills could link in. Simulated patients could be trained to respond to a myriad of situations, and synchronous presentation for eTraining or eMentoring could be implemented. Similarly, for learning test protocols and procedures, computer-simulated patients have been developed (Dzulkarnain, Wan Mhd Pandi, Wilson, Bradley, & Sapian, 2014; Heitz, Dünser, Bartneck, Grady, & Moran, 2014). These may have application in eTraining in developing countries, where accessibility to audiology programs is limited. For example, persons trained in pure-tone audiometry for hearing screening programs for school-aged children could practice on computer simulations, thus highlighting to external mentors where further training requirements lie, before allowing participation in the screening program. Araújo, Alvarenga, Urnau, Pagnossin, and Wen (2013) report the effective dissemination of infant hearing health information to community health workers (CHW) using an interactive tele-educational tool. In addition to determining that the CHWs were able to retain the information taught via distance education, they also found that they were able to apply the learned data to hypothetical situations representative of their daily activities. This highlights an important factor for consideration when developing eEducation materials, that of relevancy. In order for a clinician to benefit from a training program, there must be some significance to clinical need. Although developed countries perhaps have an obligation to disseminate expertise to aid in the creation of successful health care initiatives in the developing world, care must be taken when transferring skills to ensure usability and efficacy. For example, ABR testing for detection of acoustic neuroma requires high levels of knowledge and clinical expertise, but the likelihood is very slight that this assessment would be a priority for establishing hearing health care in an area where there are currently no audiological services.

How Hear and Say Is Delivering eTraining, eSupervision, and eMentoring to Audiologists and Listening and Spoken Language Specialists

Hear and Say is a not-for-profit, early intervention, and implantable hearing technologies organization based in Brisbane, Queensland, Australia. The organization provides services to families whose children have permanent hearing loss, through face-to-face services from six centers throughout the state of Queensland and through telepractice to families wherever they may reside, both in Australia and internationally. The Hear and Say early intervention program follows the auditory-verbal philosophy, with professionals training to become listening and spoken language specialists (LSLSs) following the principles as defined by the AG Bell Academy for Listening and Spoken Language (2014). In order to become certified by the AG Bell Academy, professionals require prior qualifications in at least one of the following disciplines: teacher of the deaf, speech pathology, or audiology. These professionals then receive additional training and mentoring for at least 3 years before being eligible to sit the certification examination of the AG Bell Academy.

Because of its expertise in this specialist field, Hear and Say has, since 2000, been providing formalized professional education and training to professionals (i.e., teachers of the deaf, speech-language pathologists, and audiologists) from throughout the world. Initially, these courses, seminars, and workshops were available only in face-to-face mode at the organization's headquarters in Brisbane. This meant, however, that professionals had to encounter huge expenses to travel from countries outside of Australia and even from within Australia, as distances are so vast that attending for a 5-day face-to-face course incurs significant time and cost to the participants. In 2010, through collaboration with Distinguished Professor Nian-Shing Chen, Hear and Say was offered the opportunity to use the Collaborative Cyber Community (CCC), a Learning Management System developed by the National Sun Yat-Sen University in Taiwan. This platform enables the use of a blended cyber model to provide education and development to professionals throughout the world.

In the Hear and Say blended model, digital (asynchronous) resources, in the form of lecture notes or PowerPoint slides with embedded narration, are uploaded to the platform for the students to view in their own time. The lectures can be made available with either restricted or unrestricted time frames. Each lecture has clearly defined learning objectives and contains a number of topic-related tasks to which students are encouraged to respond within a given time frame, with each student's responses uploaded through the CCC platform for the course instructor to access. Video recordings of, for example, assessment or teaching procedures and strategies, such as ABR testing, behavioral hearing assessment, Ling Sound Test, cochlear implant MAPping/programming, and how to implement an auditory-verbal therapy lesson with child and family, are a valuable way of sharing knowledge and expertise and as such play a significant role in the Hear and Say training courses. Videos can be loaded through the CCC platform or, if too large, then loaded through Box, Dropbox, or similar platforms. Multiple-choice examinations are able to be loaded and then marked automatically through the CCC platform, with facilities available such as allocated access time frames for the students and also restricted defined times for completion of the examination once it has been opened by individual students.

Tutorials or discussions with the students are available by using the HomeMeeting JoinNet program. This interactive Web-based system allows for synchronous and asynchronous delivery of training materials. At regular intervals, at an agreed time, a tutorial is held where all students can join a tutor in real time to discuss the task answers and any questions or concerns from the recent lectures. Students submit questions ahead of the tutorial as well as during the actual JointNet meeting. Those students who, due to time zones or other commitments, are not able to connect to the tutorial at the set time are able to access the tutorial asynchronously, as a recording function is available to record the synchronous meeting. During the tutorials, the lecturer uses spoken voice to communicate, with the students communicating back either by voice or by using the instant messaging function, which allows written communication with either selected members or all of the group. In the authors' experience, although enabling all participants to communicate via voice is optimal, this can cause difficulties with clarity, distortion, and echoing, even when all other microphones except the one in use are muted. Bandwidth available at both ends is likely to affect the quality of voice interactions. This point illustrates the importance of having expert IT support, both to assist with troubleshooting and to maximize the potential of the platform being used. The recording of the tutorial will contain all written and spoken communications. This factor needs to be considered when participants sign confidentiality agreements at the commencement of a course: The agreement needs to clearly state that all spoken and written contributions during tutorials will be recorded and available to all participants over the length of the course.

Hear and Say also works collaboratively with RIDBC Renwick Centre (which is affiliated with the University of Newcastle, New South Wales, Australia) to provide two of the four courses in their Graduate Certificate in Educational Studies (Listening and Spoken Language). These courses are provided fully online, one solely asynchronously and the other in combined synchronous and asynchronous mode. Each course consists of 13 lectures, which are all uploaded, at the beginning of a 13-week semester, to Blackboard on UoNline, the University of Newcastle's Virtual Learning Environment website. Most lectures are made available in both PDF Word format as well as PowerPoint slides with embedded voice narration. Using both formats accommodates for different learning styles of the students. Typical learning styles are one of the following three or combinations of these three: visual, auditory, and kinesthetic. Visual learners prefer images, videos, and demonstrations; they prefer to read rather than listening for long periods of time. Auditory learners learn best through listening and talking. Kinesthetic learners learn by doing, for example, by participating in group activities such as role-playing. Most learners use a combination of these three styles but may be dominant in one style. Therefore, having learning materials available in a range of formats is a valuable asset for organizations offering training and education through telepractice and demonstrates the flexibility of this model of learning.

The use of video clips to illustrate assessments or techniques adds significantly to the facilitation of transfer of knowledge. Videos are able to be loaded to the Blackboard site using a secure format, such as is offered by Vimeo, which does not allow for the videos to be further downloaded or copied. This is essential to ensure confidentiality, particularly if third parties such as client families and their children are featured on the videos. Families typically would give consent for this material to be available only to those students taking a specified course, not for general dissemination to the wider community. Videos are also a valuable way to interact with the students more personally than via written communication; for example, a video of the lecturer introducing a course and recording a video communication a few times throughout the running of the course provides a more tangible connection between lecturer and students. This is particularly beneficial for the course that does not contain any synchronous components, such as regular tutorials, as it gives a personal connection between the lecturer and students. The second course, which combines asynchronous and synchronous modes, offers synchronous multisite connections for all students and the lecturer. A tutorial could take the following form: video clip is played, demonstrating a particular assessment, technique, or case study, and then the lecturer leads the discussion, with others contributing to the conversation. This ability for synchronous interaction assists in reducing the isolation that may be experienced by students who study independently online.

When providing professional training and education through telepractice, it can be challenging for both parties to fully engage and participate. Having a combination of synchronous and asynchronous formats assists to foster better engagement for the students and more satisfaction for the lecturer. Although time zone differences make it difficult for all participants to link up in synchronous mode, the availability of recorded tutorials does go some way toward mitigating this difficulty. Significant commitment and self-motivation is required on the part of the students to ensure they access the materials in realistic time frames and set aside sufficient time both to study the content and to attend tutorials. From the lecturer's perspective, updating of materials and providing them in a range of formats to accommodate different adult learning styles is time-consuming but essential if the course is to remain relevant to the fast-changing face of today's expertise in the area of hearing impairment. Discussion groups and tutorials require preparation and planning if they are to achieve maximum benefit for all concerned, and of course the Internet connection needs to be sufficient to support the needs of all applications. Lecturers must be conscious of their speaking voice when giving tutorials, paying particular attention to accent, speed of speaking, and use of colloquialisms. As eLearning allows global access, many of the students are likely to have a different first language than that of the lecturer. In order to help assess the effectiveness of the content and to continuously improve course delivery, it is essential to obtain satisfaction feedback from the participants. At Hear and Say, surveys have been completed by participating students and lecturers over a number of years. A sample of one of these surveys is available in the Appendix. Some of the key points from these surveys are now discussed here.

Feedback from students studying these courses has indicated that the blended cyber model provides the opportunity to study content in a self-directed and independent manner while still having the opportunity to interact both with the lecturer and with other students. However, students were very much in favor of the asynchronous content being available in a variety of formats to fit the type and complexity of specific content and also to accommodate individual learning styles. PowerPoint with embedded voice narration provides a more interactive model than a written word document, with the combination of the two options being the best way to meet individual learning styles and needs. Hear and Say recently offered a "hybrid" course, where half of the content was accessed through eLearning over several weeks, with the final 2 days spent on campus. The on-campus lectures were specifically chosen for their practical components and the opportunity to hold group role-play/discussion in face-to-face mode. The feedback was that the hybrid model afforded that flexibility of accommodating different learning styles and was a way of consolidating the learning that had previously taken place through eLearning. The hybrid approach also reduced the amount of time the students were required "in person," therefore alleviating the impact on personal and work commitments, with the added benefit of less financial output for some students and their employers.

Tutorials were seen as a most important component of the eLearning courses, as they provided the opportunity for interaction both with the lecturers and also with fellow students. They were particularly beneficial for explaining complicated assessment procedures and discussing specific case studies. When small tasks were embedded in the lectures, requiring timely responses from the students, this technique was viewed as valuable in maintaining engagement of the students and also in providing a platform for the students to ask for clarification or expansion of areas of concern. These tasks and additional questions were then addressed in the tutorials, so that all students were able to benefit from the answers and queries posed by group members in the same way as students would in an on-site course. The frequency of the tutorials was also deemed to be important; for example, weekly tutorials were able to provide prompt and specific feedback about lectures studied asynchronously in the previous week. Tutorials assisted in providing an avenue for interactive discussion about the content and the opportunity to identify and have addressed areas requiring more in-depth discussion. The ability to watch or rewatch the tutorials via recording was also deemed most helpful. Feedback also reiterated the importance of the clarity of oral presentations and stated that written text to accompany the spoken tutorial was beneficial. The use of videos, as part of the asynchronous content or watched in synchronous mode, was deemed advantageous for training in the use of specific techniques or management strategies, as the visual demonstration enabled the students to follow through with practicing learned ideas in a more timely and confident manner, thus speeding up the application of their learning into their own practice. This specific feedback received from participants demonstrates the importance of seeking and then responding to feedback and in offering flexibility in the presentation modality. A positive and encouraging comment from students suggests that telepractice enables equivalent interactions, in real time, to those that occur in traditional on-site learning situations.

The terms *21st-century learning* and *21st-century skills* are used in a range of ways. The University of Melbourne, Australia, is undertaking a research project on "The Assessment and Teaching of 21st Century Skills." They describe the learning skills as including ways of thinking, ways of working, tools for working, and skills for living in the world. The two specific skills they have identified as spanning all of these areas are collaborative problem solving and Information and Communication Technology (ICT) literacy, specifically learning in digital networks (ATCS, 2014).

There has been a paradigm shift in the way students learn: from the time children begin formal schooling (and even prior to schooling) through to university study and job seeking, 21st-century technology is shaping how we learn and communicate with others. With this in mind, providing training, supervision, and mentoring through telepractice requires the application of 21st-century technology, offering a wide range of mediums for connecting people around the world.

Professionals should consider incorporating a range of these learning tools into telepractice education programs, as they enable increased connectivity between participants and more synchronous interactions. Many of these tools are commonly used by people throughout the world to connect and communicate; including them in telepractice training courses assists greatly in reducing the isolation that may exist in more traditional types of "online" learning programs. Professional learning networks (PLNs) can be established, for example, to connect a defined group of professionals who are undertaking the same professional development course. PLNs connect people via the use of established social networking sites such as Facebook, blogs, Twitter, and LinkedIn.

The Massive Open Online Course (MOOC) approach to Web-based learning has emerged in recent years, with the intent to provide open access to higher education to an unlimited number of participants. These courses use a combination of more traditional teaching resources along with interactive participant forums and cost significantly less than face-to-face higher education courses (Yuan, Powell, & Olivier, 2014). Yuan et al. (2014) note that MOOCs provide educators with new opportunities to offer more flexible forms of learning and assessment by challenging the traditional role of teacher and learner and taking advantage of digital technology. Although the original intention of MOOCs was for tertiary education, research data to date suggest that many people are using them for professional development with the result that many organizations are now providing training in this way (Hill, 2013; Yuan et al., 2014).

Hear and Say provides specialized mentoring to professionals who are undertaking further training to become LSLSs. The authors believe that the principles and techniques used for this mentoring of LSLSs would apply equally effectively to mentoring professionals in other areas of hearing health care, such as diagnostic audiology, fitting of hearing aids, and programming of cochlear implants, to name just a few. Hear and Say has five satellite centers spread across the vast state of Queensland, ranging from a 2-hour drive to more than a 2-hour airplane flight from the main center. Providing regular mentoring to junior professionals on its staff, as well as ongoing professional development and support to all clinical team members, presents challenges due to distance and the time and cost constraints associated with travel to these satellite centers. This cost has been alleviated by the use of telepractice to provide professional mentoring and support.

When commencing a mentoring relationship, it is essential for the mentor and mentee to establish a productive working relationship of mutual trust and respect. It is then necessary to ascertain the baseline skills of the mentee and for the mentor and mentee to agree on the specific skills that require targeting and how and when the mentoring will be implemented. The etiquette of mentoring also needs to be clearly established; this is even more vital when mentoring through the Internet, particularly if there are other people (such as family members or visitors) in the room with either party. It is essential that both mentor and mentee are organized, with all equipment ready and in working order, and that all paperwork is close to hand if notes are to be taken during the lesson time. Cameras and recording equipment need to be of high quality and set up in such a way as to optimally record both visual and auditory input from all relevant parties.

Until recently, Hear and Say had provided mentoring to junior clinicians who worked in regional centers by viewing a previously videotaped lesson, then providing feedback in written form or by phone, email, or Skype linkup. The disadvantage of this asynchronous telepractice model is that the feedback was provided sometimes several weeks (or at least several days) after the actual lesson took place, thus putting the feedback at risk of being less effective. Using synchronous telepractice, the mentor can now provide more timely and personal feedback to the mentee in a user-friendly interactive way. There are several options that have been used at Hear and Say to provide mentoring to professionals in regional centers, when the mentor is based at the main center in Brisbane. The following examples are taken from Listening and Spoken Language therapy lessons but could be equally well applied to other health care professional mentoring situations: (a) Using Skype, the mentor links in to observe the lesson with LSLS and parent and child in a regional center. The sound is left on at both ends, allowing the mentor to become part of the actual lesson, joining in with the activities and providing mentoring such as guiding and coaching the mentee during the actual lesson (Figure 9–1). Of course, this method requires very careful input from the mentor, as the parents will be able to hear all conversations and all parties would need to be comfortable with this situation. The advantage, though, is that mentoring can occur in real time, as if the mentor were actually in the room

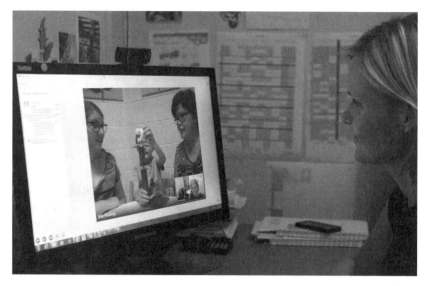

Figure 9–1. Synchronous (real-time) mentoring during a listening and spoken language session.

with the mentee and family members. Feedback regarding this method has been encouraging; children these days are very used to interacting with someone over a screen, and it can often add a very positive dimension to interactions. This method allows the mentee to adapt his or her strategies and techniques immediately to include the feedback from the mentor. (b) Use the same principle as above, but without direct input into the lesson from the mentor. Instead, the mentee uses an earpiece or Bluetooth connection to hear the mentor, thus blocking the spoken feedback from the hearing of the family members while still allowing the mentee to follow the guidance of the mentor in actual real time. This method does not disrupt the flow of the lesson or risk jeopardizing the professional-parent-child relationships within the lesson; however, it could prove challenging for the mentee to follow two conversations at the one time. (c) Use the same principle again, with the mentor observing the lesson in real time but without contributing mentoring/feedback at that time. Instead, the mentor links up again once the lesson is over, and the family has departed, to give prompt and specific feedback. This allows the mentor to observe the lesson in real time and then provide immediate feedback at the end of the lesson, while those factors requiring discussion and guidance are still fresh in people's minds, but does not risk intrusion on the flow of the lesson or on the interactions of the parent-child-professional cohort. (d) At an arranged time after completion of the lesson, the mentee, having previously recorded the lesson, connects with the mentor, for example via Lync. This allows both parties to view the recording of the lesson and for mentoring to take place while actually watching the lesson together. This is far preferable to sending a copy of the lesson for the mentor to watch on his or her own and to then supply written or oral feedback, as it allows for a collaborative viewing of the lesson and collaborative two-way critique from both mentor and mentee.

Positive reactions to real-time mentoring are that it is more time efficient to mentor a live lesson/assessment/procedure and then provide feedback either during or immediately after the event, as it allows for prompt and specific support and enables adjustments to be made immediately rather than the mentee having to wait several days or weeks for the feedback to arrive from the mentor. Although these examples are from mentoring of LSLSs, at Hear and Say, the audiologists are a vital part of a collaborative team framework. It is not unusual for the child's audiologist to join the LSLS mentor to observe a lesson. It is important for the audiologist to see how the child is functioning auditorily, as this informs further audiological adjustments that may be required to the child's amplification devices as well as providing opportunities for the audiologist to observe parent-child interactions in a nonthreatening way. Although the main center for Hear and Say has several full-time audiologists on its team, the five satellite regional centers of Hear and Say do not have full-time audiological support. When an audiologist does visit a regional center to provide services to families, this professional is usually on his or her own without the support from other members of the audiology team. Using telepractice to link in to real-time audiological procedures allows a senior audiologist in Brisbane to provide mentoring or supervision to the solo audiologist at the regional center. This is particularly valuable if an unscheduled or unexpected difficulty occurs during audiological assessment or when programing implantable hearing devices.

As discussed in previous chapters, teleaudiology is used at Hear and Say for programming cochlear implants remotely. This system is able to be used for Cochlear, MED-EL, and Advanced Bionics branded cochlear implants. This flexibility has enabled Hear and Say audiologists to provide eMentoring to a clinician in an overseas country who recently encountered her first Advanced Bionics implantee. By linking in remotely to the clinic's programming software, MAPping (or programming) is able to be provided by the Hear and Say audiologist working collaboratively with the external audiologist, using a synchronous two-way video link with audio or instant messaging capabilities. Troubleshooting and case management then occur in a team approach, with the aim to transfer clinical expertise and experience to the remote audiologist so that they will ultimately take over full case management.

Summary

Professionals are required to undertake professional development activities in order to maintain their registration and also to enable them to ensure their knowledge remains in line with current evidence-based best practice. Students, such as those in their internship phase, need to receive expert supervision but may find this difficult to access in their work location. Mentoring of professionals to develop and improve their skills in the practical application of their knowledge presents challenges for those professionals whose practice is not located near metropolitan areas or in the same location as their mentor. Telepractice provides the opportunity for professionals to access support of their choice without being constrained by restrictions such as location, time limitations, and travel costs. The authors have described some of the ways they have used telepractice to enhance their training, supervision, and mentoring programs. The uses and benefits of technology are constantly evolving; there are many diverse and exciting ways to link professionals across continents so that they can benefit from the sharing of knowledge and skills wherever they may be in the world. In this age of technology-driven innovation, professionals, whatever their level of competence and wherever they may live, have the opportunity, through telepractice, to access professional development resources and to learn and consolidate new skills. This enables them to be better equipped to improve their own practice and to facilitate optimal service to their clients.

References

AG Bell Academy for Listening and Spoken Language. (2014). *Principles of LSLS*. Retrieved June 4, 2014, from http://listeningandspoken language.org/AcademyDocument.aspx?id=563

American Speech-Language-Hearing Association. (2002). *Survey report on telepractice use among audiologists and speech-language pathologists*. Retrieved April 27, 2014, from http://www.asha.org

Araújo, E. S., Alvarenga, K. F., Urnau, D., Pagnossin, D. F., & Wen, C. L. (2013). Community health worker training for infant hearing health: Effectiveness of distance learning. *International Journal of Audiology, 52*, 636–641.

Arnold, S. A. (1985). Objective versus visual detection of the auditory brainstem response. *Ear and Hearing, 6*, 144–150.

ATCS. (2014). *About ATC21S*. Retrieved June 19, 2014, from http://atc21s.org/index.php/about

Behl, D. D., Houston, K. T., & Stredler-Brown, A. (2012). The value of a learning community to support telepractice for infants and toddlers with hearing loss. *The Volta Review, 112*, 313–328.

Crandell, C. C., & Weiner, A. (2002). Counselling competencies in audiologists: Efficacy of a distance learning course. *The Hearing Journal, 55*, 42–47.

Dzulkarnain, A. A., Wan Mhd Pandi, W. M., Wilson, W. J., Bradley, A. P., & Sapian, F. (2014). A preliminary investigation into the use of an auditory brainstem response (ABR) simulator for training audiology students in waveform analysis. *International Journal of Audiology, 53*(8), 514–521.

English, K., & Archibold, S. (2014). Measuring the effectiveness of an audiological counselling program. *International Journal of Audiology, 53*, 115–120.

Goulios, H., & Patuzzi, R. B. (2008). Audiology education and practice from an international perspective. *International Journal of Audiology, 47*, 647–664.

Heitz, A., Dünser, A., Bartneck, C., Grady, J., & Moran, C. (2014). Assessing the impact of a clinical audiology simulator on first year students. *Proceedings of the Fifteenth Australasian User Interface Conference, 150*, 11–20.

Hill, P. (2013). *MOOCs beyond professional development: Coursera's big announcement in context*. eLiterate. Retrieved May 31, 2015, from http://mfeldstein.com/moocs-beyond-professional-development-courseras-big-announcement-in-context/

Hratinski, S. (2008). A study of asynchronous and synchronous e-learning methods discovered that each support different purposes. *Educause Quarterly, 4*, 51–55.

Hutchinson, J., & Smith, P. (2014). *Facebook splurges $17.7bn on WhatsApp*. Retrieved August 5, 2015, from http://www.afr.com/technology/facebook-splurges-177bn-onwhatsapp-20140219-ixqw2

Internet World Stats. (2012). Retrieved May 11, 2014, from http://www.internetworldstats.com

Naeve-Velguth, S., Christensen, S. A., & Woods, S. (2013). Simulated patients in audiology education: Student reports. *Journal of the American Academy of Audiology, 24*, 740-746.

Page, M., Molina, M., & Jones, G. (2013). *The mobile economy*. London, UK: A. T. Kearney.

Romero, T. (2010). *Webcast vs. webinar: What's the difference?* Retrieved February 5, 2015, from http://webinarsecrets.net/webcast-vs-webinar-whats-the-difference

South Carolina CPA. (2014). *The difference between a webinar and a webcast*. Retrieved June 4, 2014, from http://www.scacpa.org/Content/ContinuingEducation/Webinars/Webcasts/Webinarvswebcast.aspx

Sutton, G., & Wood, S. (2011). *Improving the quality of newborn ABRs. Report on NHSP ABR quality improvement pilots in East of England and Greater Manchester 2009–11*. Retrieved May 11, 2014, from http://hearing.screening.nhs.uk

Vidler, M., & Parker, D. (2004). Auditory brainstem response threshold estimation: Subjective threshold estimation by experienced clinicians in a computer simulation of the clinical test. *International Journal of Audiology, 43*, 417–429.

Windmill, I. M. (2013). Academic programs, class sizes, and obstacles to growth in audiology. *Journal of the American Academy of Audiology, 24*, 417–424.

World Health Organization. (1995). *Prevention of hearing impairment. Resolution of the 48th World Health Assembly, WHA 48.9*. Retrieved May 11, 2014, from http://www.who.int/pbd/publications/wha_eb/wha48_9/en/

World Health Organization. (2013a). *Multi-country assessment of national capacity to provide hearing care.* Geneva, Switzerland: WHO Document Production Services.

World Health Organization. (2013b). *Millions of people in the world have hearing loss that can be improved or prevented.* Retrieved June 4, 2014, http://www.who.int/mediacentre/news/notes/2013/hearing_loss_20130227/en/

Yuan, L., Powell, S. & Olivier, B. (2014). *Beyond MOOCs: Sustainable online learning in institutions. Cetis white paper.* Retrieved May 31, 2015, from http://publications.cetis.org.uk/wp-content/uploads/2014/01/Beyond-MOOCs-Sustainable-Online-Learning-in-Institutions.pdf

Zolnierek, K. B. H., & DiMatteo, M. R. (2009). Physician communication and patient adherence to treatment: A meta-analysis. *Medical Care,* *47*(8), 826–834.

10

From Research to Clinical Practice: What Should We Consider?

Gabriella Constantinescu and Dimity Dornan

Key Points

- Teleaudiology has the potential to improve equity of access to services for all clients.
- Clinicians are best placed to assist with uptake of teleaudiology into clinical practice as they interpret and adopt research findings into clinical practice and by themselves undertaking research studies.
- A strong relationship must be established between research and clinical practice.

In this era of technology driving innovation, we are witnessing a transformational change in the audiology profession. Modern digital hearing devices are revolutionizing hearing for clients, and for clinicians, applications are making the diagnosis and treatment of hearing loss and the delivery of services more efficient and user-friendly and allowing for better outcomes for clients. Like other health disciplines, telepractice has emerged as a frontrunner in audiology with the potential to address inequity issues that are still faced for clients, particularly access to services. Research studies in teleaudiology are still in their infancy, and as the field continues to grow, so too will our knowledge of telepractice benefits for clients and organizations, as well as the potential for long-term uptake into clinical services and sustainability. Translational research, where processes and findings are moved from laboratory-based studies to clinical settings (Wikipedia, 2014), will ultimately facilitate the uptake and sustainability of teleaudiology. Clinicians are best placed to aid translational research as they interpret and adopt research findings into clinical practice and by themselves undertaking research studies to fill knowledge gaps that meet the needs of their clients directly. Therefore, a strong relationship must be established between research and clinical practice. Clinicians must have an awareness of how to interpret studies in the context of evidence-based research, draw out implications for clinical practice, and determine possible future research needs that will assist with the long-term uptake and sustainability of telepractice. This chapter guides clinicians in this process by presenting an overview of evidence-based practice and the levels of evidence in research studies, examples of how research outcomes from various levels of evidence can be relevant to clinical practice, suggestions for future research needs in building the evidence base for telepractice, and a guide for clinicians to assist with undertaking research studies.

Evidence-Based Practice

Evidence-based practice is a term commonly used in both the research and clinical settings. The American Speech-Language-Hearing Association (ASHA, 2014a) defines evidence-based practice as "the integration of: (a) clinical expertise/expert opinion, (b) external scientific evidence, and (c) client/patient/caregiver values to provide high-quality services reflecting the interests, values, needs, and choices of the individuals we serve." Evidence-based practice in the clinical setting ensures that intervention is effective. The principles of evidence-based practice and their relationship to each other are represented in Figure 10–1.

Research studies help to inform evidence-based practice. Studies that are well designed and employing large participant numbers are likely to answer the research and clinical ques-

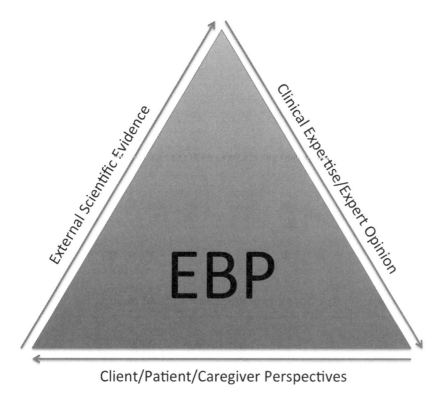

Client/Patient/Caregiver Perspectives

Figure 10–1. Relationship between principles in evidence-based practice. Adapted from ASHA (2014a).

tions such as the effectiveness of teleaudiology for the delivery of specific services. When studies consistently demonstrate the effectiveness of an intervention, that intervention can be viewed as evidence based (Rhoades, 2010).

Levels of Evidence

Studies are classified according to different levels of research evidence, and an example of a commonly used classification system is presented in Table 10–1. When looking at research outcomes and implications for practice, clinicians need to consider the level of evidence of the studies. The higher the level,

Table 10–1. Levels of Research Evidence

Ia	Ib	IIa	IIb	III	IV
Well-designed meta-analysis of >1 randomized controlled trial	Well-designed randomized controlled study	Well-designed controlled study without randomization	Well-designed quasi-experimental study	Well-designed nonexperimental studies (i.e., correlational and case studies)	Expert committee report, consensus conference, clinical experience of respected authorities

Source: Adapted from ASHA (2014b).

the more likely the studies are evidence based, are reliable, have reduced bias and subjectivity, and will answer research and clinical questions.

Using the classification system, Level I evidence relates to well-designed, randomized controlled trials involving large participant numbers with a minimum of 30 participants allocated to each group. At this level, participants are ideally matched on a number of variables that may impact outcomes (e.g., matched for age at diagnosis of the hearing loss, type and severity of the hearing loss, type of amplification, age at fitting of amplification, age at intervention). Randomization of participants helps to eliminate bias and ensures that outcomes reflect the specific assessment or treatment effects (e.g., remote cochlear implant mapping via teleaudiology is providing comparable outcomes to traditional face-to-face mapping rather than outcomes relating to participant differences in age or proficiency of cochlear implant use). Level I studies include a control group for comparison and may also have the added scientific rigor of blinding, where, for example, the assessors are unaware of the treatment environment allocated to the participant (experimental or control) and/ or the treatment outcomes (where applicable).

Level II evidence represents well-designed, nonrandomized studies. These studies follow the progress of participants over time in order to examine particular outcomes and may involve a control group for comparison (e.g., children with typical hearing of the same age; participants receiving treatment in the control condition). Level III evidence involves nonexperimental research designs such as retrospective studies, case studies, or questionnaires. Level IV is the lowest level of evidence and provides very little indication of assessment or treatment success. Examples of Level IV studies include group judgements or expert opinions of performance (ASHA, 2014b; Dornan, Hickson, Murdoch, & Houston, 2008; Eriks-Brophy, 2004; Rhoades, 2006).

Applying Research Outcomes to Clinical Practice

It is important for clinicians to be aware that studies across the different levels of evidence can be useful and applicable to clinical practice. This section demonstrates clinical applicability by providing some examples of research studies with Level I to Level III evidence and how outcomes can be relevant to clinical practice. Directions for future research that could strengthen the level of evidence of the studies and their clinical applicability are also suggested.

Level I Studies

Andersson, Strömgren, Ström, and Lyttkens (2002) conducted a randomized controlled trial to investigate the benefits of an Internet-based self-help cognitive behavior therapy program for tinnitus. In this study, 117 participants were randomly assigned to either cognitive behavior therapy ($n = 53$) or a control group on a waiting list ($n = 64$). All aspects of the program were accessed via the Internet (e.g., modules and homework assignments), and the investigators were in email contact with the participants to instruct about the modules and to answer any questions. Compared to the controls, the treatment group made significant improvements in their self-rated tinnitus problems and psychological complaints at the completion of the study and at 1-year follow-up. The improvements were also clinically significant for 28% of the treatment group. Clinical implications: The authors suggested that this form of Internet-based self-help program would be beneficial as a complementary service to traditional tinnitus management in the clinic. This type of program may be an option for clinicians wanting to refer their clients. However, the high dropout or delayed response rate (42%) would suggest that it may not be suited to all clients. Some of the areas that participants found challenging and impacted treatment completion included participant time constraints and lack of a quiet home environment to complete the modules in, as well as the fast pace, demand, and impersonal nature of the program. Further research: Studies looking at the impact of the above factors on treatment completion as well as participant motivation would allow for better profiling of clients who would most likely benefit from this type of Internet-based treatment. Follow-up beyond 1 year posttreatment would also provide a greater reflection of the long-term success of the program. These findings would be useful when counseling clients about the potential treatment benefits.

Level II Studies

Swanepoel, Mngemane, Molemong, Mkwanazi, and Tutshini (2010) studied the reliability, accuracy, and efficiency of teleaudiometry using 30 participants with typical hearing and 8 participants with hearing loss. Test-retest reliability was performed with the group of participants with typical hearing by repeating testing using both the conventional manual audiometer and the auto-mated teleaudiometer. The authors found teleaudiometry to be time-efficient, reliable, and accurate, with comparable thresholds between the two environments. A high percentage (63%) of par-ticipants with typical hearing also preferred teleaudiometry to standard practice. Clinical implications: The outcomes suggested that teleaudiometry may be considered an appropriate service delivery option for performing hearing assessments in real time. Further research: Studies using larger participant numbers, par-ticularly those participants with differing levels of hearing loss and ages, will add to the knowledge base of the applicability of teleaudiometry in the clinical setting. User satisfaction (client and clinician) should also be examined as this factor may impact uptake (only rated for participants with typical hearing in the study). The authors acknowledged that further investigations of teleaudiometry in settings without the use of soundproof booths would indicate the functionality of this type of assessment for use in rural and remote areas or where access to traditional audiology services is limited.

Givens and colleagues (2003) also investigated the use of teleaudiometry using 31 university students and staff with both hearing loss and typical hearing. Their auditory thresholds were assessed using a conventional and teleaudiometry system. In this double-blinded study, the participants were unaware of which audiometer was being used in the assessments, and the audi-ologists were unaware of previous testing results. The study demonstrated the feasibility of teleaudiometry with substantial agreement between results using the conventional and tele-audiometry systems. Clinical implications: The study findings suggested that teleaudiometry may be a feasible method for remote hearing assessments conducted in real time. The detailed description of the teleaudiometry system will be useful for cli-nicians wishing to replicate the study and for potential clinical uptake. Further research: Similar to the study by Swanepoel et al.

(2010), extending the research to include greater participant numbers with hearing loss and of various ages will provide further information about applicability to the clinical setting. A randomized controlled trial where both participants and audiologists are randomized to the assessment environment would also validate teleaudiometry and ensure a Level I evidence study.

Eikelboom, Mbao, Coates, Atlas, and Gallop (2005) looked at the otolaryngologist's ability to assess and provide management advice about the child's ear condition using information from all of teleotoscopy, audiometry, tympanometry, and clinical history. Here, 66 children from remote communities in Australia were assessed face-to-face by the specialist, who then also later reassessed the children using the digital images captured at the time of face-to-face assessment. Significant agreement was found between the two environments for clinically relevant observations, diagnoses, review, and referral recommendations. Clinical implications: The study demonstrated the validity of teleotoscopy in the clinical setting. The model and outcomes may be relevant for other clinicians working in similar settings. The authors noted that the comprehensive assessment battery comprising teleotoscopy, audiometry, tympanometry data, and clinical history allowed for the accurate diagnosis and clinical management of the clients. Further research: It would be interesting to look at study outcomes where other health professionals or support personnel conduct the teleotoscopy (the current study used an experienced video-otoscopist), as this is more likely to occur in clinical practice. The outcomes of these studies and recommendations for practice would further assist with uptake of telepractice in this setting.

Ribera (2005) investigated the interjudge reliability and validity of conducting the Hearing in Noise Test via telepractice. For this study, 20 university students were assessed in both the face-to-face and remote environment. The study showed high reliability and validity for the telepractice application. Clinical implications: The validation outcomes suggested that the Hearing in Noise Test may be considered appropriate for use via telepractice. Further research: As this study was conducted using young adults with typical hearing (aged between 18 and 30 years) and with audiologists administering the assessments, the authors recognized the need for future studies including participants with hearing loss of varying ages and involving technicians or aides to support the assessments. Such studies would provide further information about the usability and uptake of the Hearing in Noise Test via telepractice.

Level III Studies

This earlier study by Eikelboom, Atlas, Mbao, and Gallop (2002) presented details on the planning, design, development, and implementation of a teleotoscopy system. Real-time and store-and-forward of still images were able to be examined by the otolaryngologist, and this approach forms part of a clinical service in a remote Australian community. Clinical implications: The authors outlined the importance of training of rural health care workers delivering the sessions so that optimal examinations and assessments could be made by specialists. Training may need to be considered for other services providing telepractice where health professionals or support personnel other than audiologists are involved. Further research: Combining the level of detail on planning, design, development, and implementation of teleotoscopy with objective data on the validity of the approach, such as with the later Eikelboom et al. (2005) study, would provide further indication of the success of teleotoscopy in this setting.

Eikelboom and Atlas (2005) also surveyed 116 patients in four audiology centers to learn about their regular face-to-face appointments (including travel, distance, time, and waiting time), willingness to have a telemedicine appointment if that was available (specific service type not specified), and use of the Internet for health matters. Potential willingness to use telemedicine was associated with perceived reduced waiting time and cost, prior understanding of telemedicine and the use of the Internet for health matters, and, in some instances, age and gender (women under 55 years were more willing to use telemedicine). Unwillingness was associated with preferring the face-to-face appointments. Clinical implications: Client familiarity with the concept of telepractice and exposure to telepractice applications may need to be considered when implementing a telepractice service as this may promote patient willingness and uptake. Clinicians may need to consider client need on a case-by-case basis. Further research: A follow-up survey once the teleaudiology service is implemented would allow for a more representative look at actual willingness and barriers to service uptake from the level of the client. Comparison of time and cost of telepractice to traditional face-to-face service from the client and organizational level would also provide further indication of potential uptake and sustainability.

Rushbrooke (2012) administered a satisfaction survey in addition to conducting an evaluation of telemapping. The children with cochlear implants ($n = 20$), their parents ($n = 24$), and clinicians conducting the telemapping ($n = 6$) rated their level of satisfaction with the procedure. All participant groups reported high levels of satisfaction with the audio and video quality and time taken to complete the sessions, sound quality of the MAPs (rated by the children with cochlear implants), usefulness, and overall satisfaction with telemapping. The children with cochlear implants and their parents felt that a telemapping service would be beneficial to them and their family as it would reduce travel time to the clinic. The clinicians were also very confident with the mapping results and reported the online equipment to be easy to use. Clinical implications: The high levels of satisfaction with telemapping reported by the children, parents, and clinicians indicated the potential for use in clinical practice. Some delays in the audio were occasionally noted by participants during the sessions, and such issues may need to be taken into account when delivering the service. Furthermore, the author noted that additional considerations may be necessary when working with very young children who require immediate stimulus responses as part of testing. Parent feedback also suggested that this type of service may assist not only families in regional and remote areas but also those older children/young adults with school or work demands on their time and impacting availability to access services, as well as those children only requiring quick troubleshooting of devices. Further research: As the majority of children involved in the study were from metropolitan areas, it would be important to replicate the satisfaction study with families from rural and remote areas to look at their level of satisfaction and potential benefit from the service, as well as for those older children/young adults who could benefit from this type of service delivery. As mentioned earlier, a cost-benefit analysis from the level of the client and organization would also be useful in looking at the potential long-term sustainability of such a service.

Increasing the Evidence Base in Teleaudiology and the Role Clinicians Can Play

The examples provided in this chapter have highlighted how study findings from various levels of evidence can have clinical relevance. Teleaudiology, although still emerging, is showing promise as a viable alternate or additional service delivery model for improving client equity of service access. Further research will only continue to strengthen the evidence base and support clinical uptake. To ensure this, a greater number of studies of the highest levels of evidence, that are longitudinal in nature, and employing high participant numbers need to be undertaken. See http://www.consort-statement.org/ for the Consort 2010 Checklist and Flow Diagram. These studies should be encouraged in both the research and clinical settings. Some considerations when undertaking evidence-based research that may further assist with translation into clinical practice are outlined in the following box.

A Telepractice Service Developed to Address Clinical Need

Clinicians are best placed to facilitate the process of evidence-based research and relevance of research to the clinical setting. Some considerations to facilitate the process of translational research are outlined in the following box. The example provided here highlights the second suggestion in the box where a telepractice service was developed to address a specific need, with direct relevance to the clinical setting.

Hear and Say is an early intervention auditory-verbal therapy and pediatric implantable technologies center in Queensland, Australia, with a main center in Brisbane, and five regional centers throughout Queensland. The audiology program provides diagnostic services for both nonenrolled and enrolled children with hearing loss in the early intervention program, candidacy

---

Considerations When Undertaking Evidence-Based Research and Translation to Clinical Practice

- Rigorous study designs focusing on Level I and II studies and longitudinal in nature (where applicable)
- Large participant numbers of differing levels of hearing loss and ages to best represent the standard clinical population
- Assessment and treatment settings realistic of telepractice environment (i.e., without use of soundproof booths)
- Comprehensive evaluation of user satisfaction (client and clinician)
- Time and cost comparisons between telepractice and traditional service (client and organization)
- Enough detail on planning, design, development, and implementation to assist with study replication and uptake
- Use of health professionals and support personnel to conduct assessments to best represent telepractice setting
- Evaluation of client factors that may impact telepractice outcomes
- Clinical implications of studies, translation into clinical practice, and future directions clearly stated to guide further research and uptake
- Strategies provided for clinicians to assist with service delivery
- Collaborating with other research and clinical centers to combine smaller studies into large-scale studies
- Replicating studies in different settings to determine clinical applicability
- Detailing any licensing, reimbursement, and funding requirements (where applicable) to assist with long-term sustainability

---

assessment up to 17 years of age for implantable technologies (range of cochlear and middle ear implants), and all of life mapping of implantable technologies. There are currently 183 children and young adults accessing the audiology program, and approximately 60% of them reside outside of metropolitan Brisbane. These families were previously challenged by the distance, time, travel, and cost of accessing the audiology program offered in Brisbane. In addition, the same issues from an organizational level were making it increasingly difficult for clinicians to travel on a six-monthly or yearly basis to the regional centers to offer services as the alternative option to meeting client need. In response to the increased need for equitable access to the mapping service for all children at Hear and Say, and a more efficient organizational model of service delivery, a teleaudiology research project was undertaken in collaboration with the University of Queensland and the HEARing Cooperative Research Centre. The scope of this project was to develop and validate a telemapping application for use within the clinical setting (Rushbrooke, 2012). Forty participants aged between 5 and 23 years took part in this Level II study and were broadly representative of the clinical population accessing the audiology program at Hear and Say. Participants were mapped in both the face-to-face and remote environments by two clinicians, and the order of mapping was randomized. In the face-to-face environment, the clinician in the same room as the participant conducted the session, and the remote clinician was silent. In the remote assessment, the remote clinician interacted with the participant via videoconferencing, and the clinician in the same room acted as a support personnel or facilitator where needed. Clinicians were alternated to the assessment environment and blinded to the mapping level obtained in the other environment. For this study, a custom-made videoconferencing system allowed for real-time interaction between the participant and clinician, as well as the ability for the clinician to also operate the cochlear implant programming software remotely. The results showed the validity of the telemapping system with no significant differences between electrode current level and speech perception measures in the face-to-face and remote conditions (Rushbrooke, 2012). High satisfaction with telemaping from the level of the child, parent, and clinician was also obtained (Rushbrooke, 2012).

Following validation, the telemapping system was able to be integrated as part of Hear and Say's eAudiology program. The model of service delivery established here included having telemapping systems onsite at each regional center and the onsite auditory-verbal therapist or audiologist (where applicable) being the support personnel or facilitator for the clinician conducting the assessment in Brisbane, as well as the auditory-verbal therapists taking along the telemapping systems on their yearly remote visits to the children enrolled in the auditory-verbal therapy early intervention. Here, the auditory-verbal therapists are able to be the support personnel for the audiology assessments conducted in the home, in a school setting, or at a local audiology center with access to a soundproof booth (where applicable). Guidelines and instructions for equipment use (e.g., setup, assessment, troubleshooting) were established for the eAudiology program and included considerations based on the research findings (e.g., the need to monitor user satisfaction from the level of the clinician, child and family, and support personnel or facilitator; the need for the clinician to liaise with the auditory-verbal therapist and family on the child's listening ability and spoken language progress to ensure the telemapping was successful). All audiologists and auditory-verbal therapists were provided with hands-on training prior to the rollout of the eAudiology program to assist with proficiency of use and uptake.

Since rollout, feedback on the eAudiology program has been positive from staff, children, and their families, and a follow-up satisfaction study postimplementation of the program is in preparation. Future research is also being planned based on clinical direction to extend the services offered as part of the eAudiology program to include speech perception testing and teleaudiometry as part of a comprehensive service. A further cost-benefit analysis would also provide a comprehensive measure of the cost and time savings, which are now anecdotally being reported by families as the eAudiology program allows access to services within their local community, and at the organizational level due to the reduced need for clinician travel to regional centers. The features of the telemapping system, including its portability, ease of use, privacy option (virtual private network available), and high-quality videoconferencing, have met the organizational requirements and aided clinical uptake and satisfaction. These features, along with the ability of the technology to further support the extension of audiology services as part of the future eAudiology program, will aid the long-term sustainability of the eAudiology program.

Clinicians as Drivers for Translational Research

- Interpreting studies in the context of evidence-based research, drawing out implications for clinical practice, and determining future needs
- Determining gaps in existing research, identifying areas of clinical need, and formulating research questions that are directly relevant to the clinical context
- Collaborating with universities to undertaking evidence-based research based on Level I and II studies
- Trialing and implementing research outcomes into clinical practice and providing feedback and future directions
- Building on existing research projects and developing novel projects
- Encouraging a culture of research and evaluation in clinical practice
- Collaborating with other clinicians and researchers
- Clinicians becoming lifelong learners where they are continually increasing their knowledge and keeping up to date with current research
- Advocating for services at the community, institutional, and government levels

---

Teleaudiology has the potential to improve access to services for all clients irrespective of their geographic location. Clinicians can drive this change and facilitate uptake of teleaudiology by bridging the gap between research and clinical practice. This is an exciting pioneering time for the profession.

References

American Speech-Language-Hearing Association. (2014a). *Introduction to evidence-based practice: What it is (and what it isn't)*. Retrieved May 12, 2014, from http://www.asha.org/Members/ebp/intro/
American Speech-Language-Hearing Association. (2014b). *Steps in the process of evidence-based practice: Step 3. Assessing the evidence.*

Retrieved May 12, 2014, from http://www.asha.org/members/ebp/assessing.htm

Andersson, G., Strömgren, T., Ström, L., & Lyttkens, L. (2002). Randomized controlled trial of Internet-based cognitive behavior therapy for distress associated with tinnitus. *Psychosomatic Medicine, 64*, 810–816.

Dornan, D., Hickson, L., Murdoch, B., & Houston, T. (2008). Speech and language outcomes for children with hearing loss educated in auditory-verbal therapy programs: A review of the evidence. *Communicative Disorders Review, 2*(3–4), 157–172.

Eikelboom, R., & Atlas, M. (2005). Attitude to telemedicine, and willingness to use it, in audiology patients. *Journal of Telemedicine and Telecare, 11*(Suppl. 2), 22–25.

Eikelboom, R., Atlas, M., Mbao, M., & Gallop, M. (2002). Tele-otology: Planning, design, development and implementation. *Journal of Telemedicine and Telecare, 8*(Suppl. 3), 14–17.

Eikelboom, R., Mbao, M., Coates, H., Atlas, M., & Gallop, M. (2005). Validation of tele-otology to diagnose ear disease in children. *International Journal of Pediatric Otorhinolaryngology, 69*, 739–744.

Eriks-Brophy, A. (2004). Outcomes of auditory-verbal therapy: A review of the evidence and a call for action. *Volta Review, 104*(1), 21–35.

Givens, G., Blanarovich, A., Murphy, T., Simmons, S., Blanch, D., & Elangovan, S. (2003). Internet-based tele-audiometry system for the assessment of hearing: A pilot study. *Telemedicine Journal of e-Health, 9*(4), 375–378.

Rhoades, E. A. (2010). Evidence-based auditory-verbal practice. In E. A. Rhoades & J. Duncan (Eds.), *Auditory-verbal practice: Toward a family centred approach* (pp. 23–51). Springfield, IL: Charles C Thomas.

Rhoades, E. A. (2006). Research outcomes of auditory-verbal intervention: Is the approach justified? *Deafness Education International, 8*(3), 129–143.

Ribera, J. (2005). Interjudge reliability and validation of telehealth applications of the Hearing in Noise Test. *Seminars in Hearing, 26*, 13–18.

Rushbrooke, E. (2012). *Remote MAPping for children with cochlear implants* (Unpublished master's thesis). Brisbane, Australia: The University of Queensland.

Swanepoel, D., Mngemane, S., Molemong, S., Mkwanazi, H., & Tutshini, S. (2010). Hearing assessment: Reliability, accuracy, and efficiency of automated audiometry. *Telemedicine and e-Health, 16*(5), 557–563.

Wikipedia. (2014). *Translational research*. Retrieved May 12, 2014, from http://en.wikipedia.org/wiki/Translational_research

11

Future Directions in Teleaudiology

De Wet Swanepoel and Robert H. Eikelboom

Key Points

- The birth and development of audiology as a profession has always been closely linked to discoveries in technology.
- Teleaudiology is considered one of the promising ways to address the increasing demand for ear and hearing health care services globally.
- Technology and connectivity advances are ensuring teleaudiology is becoming an increasingly feasible way to provide access to care.
- Personal computing devices, global connectivity, and automation are important future drivers that will impact the way teleaudiology services develop.
- Ear and hearing mHealth will be a major area of development in the future.
- Decentralization of audiology to meet the growing need for services will be a key emphasis of teleaudiology.
- The audiology profession should harness the benefits of teleaudiology to maximize the reach and impact of our limited audiological resources.

The field of telehealth has emerged and continues to develop in the sphere of evolving technologies in an increasingly connected world. It is not a new field in and of itself but is a health delivery conduit utilizing technology and connectivity to provide traditional health services, from prevention to rehabilitation, in novel and sometimes untraditional ways. It is this novelty and change inherent to telehealth that often leads to uncertainty and hesitancy to explore possible patient and clinician benefits. This is also true in audiology where new technologies or novel paradigms have traditionally been resisted, at least initially.

Even the most fundamental assessment instrument to the audiologist, the pure-tone audiometer, was once a novel instrument resisted by many. In 1922, Dr. Max Goldstein said the following about the pure-tone audiometer: "I have not found anything in these tests, as yet, that seems to be of any assistance . . . I plead guilty of being a mere otologist. The more I see of the audiometer the more respect I have for the tuning fork and Galton Whistle" (Transactions of the American Otological Society, 1922). Of course, much of the initial skepticism of new technologies or novel paradigms is an important part of ensuring our practices are based on evidence. Even in the presence of evidence, however, change is still often a difficult and painful process.

Future change in audiological service delivery is inevitable, especially with mounting global pressures on ear and hearing health care. Teleaudiology will play an important role as part of service delivery models in the future. For the profession of audiology, it is important to take the lead in directing the way in which teleaudiology can be utilized to support our professional services to a growing number of persons in an accountable and relevant manner.

Access to Care—Directing the Teleaudiology Future

The pervasive and prevalent nature of hearing loss along with a global shortage in available ear and hearing health care providers significantly restricts access to care. In a world where these pressures are real and mounting, teleaudiology offers a potential way to provide services to the growing number of patients with hearing loss within the context of limited and inequitably distributed professional resources.

Demand for Ear and Hearing Health Care

Major global health care challenges currently relate to issues of access, equity, quality, and cost-effectiveness (World Health Organization [WHO], 2010). On a global scale, ear and hearing health care services are faced with these same challenges. Hearing loss is a significant global health care burden expected to increase in coming years with few trained health care providers to serve this population. Current estimates indicate that 5.3% of the world population—360 million people—have a permanent disabling hearing loss (WHO, 2013a). Furthermore, these numbers are expected to increase significantly in coming decades due to the steadily increasing average life expectancies globally. Since 1990, average life expectancy has increased from 64 to 68 years in 2009 with an increase from 76 to 80 years in high-income countries (WHO, 2011). Prevalence of age-related hearing loss increases exponentially above 60 years of age, which means an unmatched growth in hearing loss prevalence in the foreseeable future (Swanepoel, Eikelboom, Hunter, Friedland, & Atlas, 2013). As a result, adult-onset hearing loss is projected to be the seventh most significant contributor to the global burden of disease (WHO, 2008).

The pressure of an increasingly widespread burden of hearing loss globally is already, and will continue to be, a major driver for the utilization of telehealth as a way to reach more patients with disabling hearing loss in a more cost-effective manner. This pressure is all the more pressing in light of the grave global shortage of ear and hearing health professionals.

Professional Capacity to Deliver Ear and Hearing Health Care

An increase in hearing loss prevalence means a higher demand on current ear and hearing health care services globally. This will strain the existing shortage of hearing health care professionals, with regions such as sub-Saharan Africa and Southeast Asia typically presenting with less than one audiologist for every million people (Fagan & Jacobs, 2009; WHO, 2013b). With such inequitable distributions of ear and hearing health care providers, it is unsurprising that an estimated 80% of persons with hearing loss are unable to access required services, because they reside in developing countries (Fagan & Jacobs, 2009; Goulios & Patuzzi, 2008; WHO, 2006).

The shortage of hearing health services is not a problem restricted to developing countries. In a country such as the United States, for example, there is a major capacity shortage in respect to the need for hearing evaluations and the capacity of the available audiological workforce. Estimates have indicated that there was an annual shortfall of 8 million audiograms in the year 2000, projected to increase to 15 million by 2050 (Margolis & Morgan, 2008). More recent analyses of demand for audiologists in relation to current and projected growth rate for new graduates suggest a growing mismatch between the demand for audiological services and capacity to deliver these (Windmill & Freeman, 2013). These estimates propose that an increase of 50% in terms of new audiology graduates and a lowering of the attrition rate to 20% is required immediately to meet the demand. Apart from general shortages in professionals, there are also specific underserved regions that persist in developed countries such as Canada, Australia, and parts of Scandinavia due to traveling distances and geographical and weather obstacles.

There is no short-term answer to sufficiently increase the number of qualified providers required to deliver ear and hearing health services to those with disabling hearing loss around the world. This poses a major barrier to any efforts that aim to address or alleviate the increasing burden of disabling hearing loss around the world. The shortage and inequitable distribution of required human resources in ear and hearing health is another major driver for telehealth as a way to open up access to care (Swanepoel, Clark, et al., 2010; Swanepoel, Olusanya, & Mars, 2010).

Future Technology Drivers for Teleaudiology

The field of audiology has always been closely linked to developments in technology. The technological breakthrough by

Alexander Graham Bell with the invention of the telephone, for example, was an important driver for the simultaneous development of the audiometer in various parts of the world (Mester & Stephens, 1984). This was one of the early seeds for the emergence of audiology as a profession in its own right. The other technological developments that were germinal to audiology were the advances in hearing aid technology, starting with carbon hearing aids at the turn of the 19th century, followed by vacuum-tube hearing aids and then transistor hearing aids that allowed more practicable amplification solutions to those identified with hearing loss. Technological advances have been driving the profession of audiology since its inception with new test methods and procedures employed as technologies have enabled more precise measurement. Teleaudiology is no different. It is this growth in technology and connectivity that is now impacting audiological practice and driving the inclusion of telehealth methods to serve patients with hearing loss (Clark & Swanepoel, 2014; Swanepoel, Clark, et al., 2010). Some of the main future technology drivers underlying growth in teleaudiology are briefly considered below.

Personal Technology Revolution

Technologies are becoming increasingly personal, mobile, and affordable. Mobile devices such as smartphones, tablets, and phablets are giving users advanced computer processing abilities in the palm of their hands (Clark & Swanepoel, 2014). These technologies are reaching a rapidly increasing world population. In 2011, an estimated 1.6 billion personal computers were in use around the world compared to 1.8 billion mobile handsets sold in 2011 alone (Minges, 2012). Sales in smartphones are increasing as low-cost units proliferate for developing world markets. From 2011 to 2013, the number of units sold increased by 200% with 1.4 billion smartphones sold at the end of 2013 (ABI Research, 2013). In line with these trends, personal computing devices will soon be universally available not only in the developed world but in developing world regions. This means an important door is opening up for personalized telehealth access to populations previously cut off from health services. Personal devices like smartphones incorporate a host of features and internal sensors (e.g., sensors in cameras, gyroscopes, accelerometers, and Global Positioning Systems [GPS]), which open up unique opportunities for personalized health monitoring, screening, and even assessments and intervention (Clark & Swanepoel, 2014). These tools are already being incorporated for teleaudiology purposes (Swanepoel, Myburgh, Howe, Mahomed, & Eikelboom, 2014) but will greatly impact the way in which services are provided into the future. It is likely that patient services will incorporate these technologies at various levels from screening right through to counseling.

Mobile Connectivity Revolution

Telehealth requires reliable Internet connectivity as a prerequisite for the provision of services. This traditionally has been one of the major barriers to telehealth implementation in developing world regions, such as sub-Saharan Africa, where fixed-line Internet is extremely uncommon (Swanepoel, Olusanya, & Mars, 2010). In the past few years, however, a mobile revolution has emerged to impact the way in which modern society communicates and exchanges information (Kelly & Minges, 2012; Swanepoel, 2014). In 2010, 90% of the world population had access to a mobile cell signal compared to 61% in 2003. It is estimated that as from 2014, there were more mobile subscriptions worldwide than people. Everywhere cellular networks are available, Internet connectivity becomes possible, and in developing countries, mobile phones are increasingly being employed to access the Internet. Although mobile data costs can still be prohibitively high, they have become more affordable over time with mobile operators also starting to open up their networks to allow for subsidized or zero-rated data charges for health applications in developing countries. This mobile revolution is at the start of its growth curve, and as a result, it will have a major impact on ear and hearing health care delivery in the future.

Automation for Efficiency and Reach

Another important driver for teleaudiology is the incorporation of automation in audiological procedures. Advances in computer technology are making automation easier, and as a result, there has been increasing interest in recent years to maximize audiological human resource efficiency through automation (Margolis, Glasberg, Creeke, & Moore, 2010; Swanepoel, Mngemane, Molemong, Mkwanazi, & Tutshini, 2010). Asynchronous or store-and-forward telehealth models can be powerful tools when automated screening and diagnostic measures are facilitated in remote or underserved areas with audiologists being able to remotely assess and interpret test results toward effective interventions. Examples of automated testing include diagnostic pure-tone audiometry, which a recent meta-analysis indicated to be equally accurate and reliable compared to the gold standard of manual audiometry (Mahomed, Swanepoel, Eikelboom, & Soer, 2013). Limitations acknowledged by this study did include limited evidence for bone conduction audiometry, for patients with various degrees and types of hearing loss, and for difficult-to-test populations (Mahomed et al., 2013). Newer computer-operated audiometric technologies have incorporated the use of automation alongside other advanced features such as noise monitoring and ambient noise attenuation (insert earphone use covered by circumaural earcups) to make these types of teleaudiology services feasible (Maclennan-Smith, Swanepoel, & Hall, 2013; Swanepoel, Maclennan-Smith, & Hall, 2013).

The Future of Teleaudiology: Examples

Ear and Hearing mHealth

In keeping with the rapid pace of technological developments, telehealth is a dynamic and rapidly changing health care delivery medium. The future of teleaudiology is likely to follow the trends in technology and connectivity discussed above. This is also reflected by the continuous emergence of new terminology to describe different forms of health care provision using information and communication technologies (Fatehi & Wootton, 2012). One such area of current interest and rapid growth and development is mobile health (mHealth), often seen as a subset of eHealth but relating to the use of mobile phone technologies to promote, provide, and monitor health care services (Kelly & Minges, 2012). This field is particularly appealing with the widespread penetration of mobile phones and cellular network reception globally, but particularly in underserved developing countries (Kelly & Minges, 2012).

A 2013 review reported that there are already more than 15,000 health care applications available for mobile devices (Fiordelli, Diviani, & Schulz, 2013). Evidence in support of these applications in clinical practice is largely unavailable, but mHealth initiatives are a priority area with governments in developing countries employing them for public health services such as maternal and child health. For ear and hearing health care, numerous smartphone applications are available to conduct a range of audiological services, such as hearing assessments (e.g., pure-tone audiometry, speech audiometry), viewing the external ear canal, ambient noise level measurements, programming hearing aids, and/or even functioning as a hearing aid (Figure 11–1). Although there are significant challenges when equipment calibration is not controlled, these personal computing technologies have considerable potential (Foulad, Bui, & Djalilian, 2013; Handzel et al., 2013; Khoza-Shangase & Kassner, 2013). A recent application was reported, however, to allow for accurate objective calibration of an entry-level smartphone and off-the-shelf headphone for hearing screening (Swanepoel et al., 2014). The application also incorporates the smartphone touch screen as an easy user-friendly interface with automated test sequences that make screening possible by teachers, community health care workers, or volunteers with almost no training requirements. It also utilizes the phone microphone to monitor background noise for quality control and stores rich data for uploading to a cloud-based server from where that data can be monitored (Swanepoel et al., 2014).

mHealth ear and hearing solutions will continue to proliferate and impact audiological care. In many cases, they are

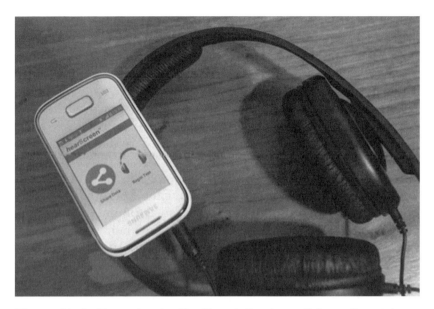

Figure 11–1. Example of mHealth solution in audiology. Smartphone application (hearScreen) for hearing screening that allows for accurate calibration and noise monitoring during tests. Application also uploads all data to a cloud-based server for data management and surveillance.

already being utilized to provide an access point for services that include information/education, screening, and possibly also diagnosis and interventions. It is important to note, however, that the majority of hearing health applications available have not been independently validated. Similarly, many of those apps that have been validated are not widely available. Evidence-based practice must direct the use of mHealth for ear and hearing health care in the future.

Decentralization of Audiological Services

Advances in technologies are offering greater possibilities, within a telehealth framework, to address the overwhelming need for audiological services to the majority of the world population. The technologies require rethinking existing audiological models of service delivery to allow patients to benefit from increased access to care. Historically, audiological services have been predominantly based in specialized health care centers or clinics because of the stringent requirements for audiological testing within sound-treated environments. As a result, audiology typically has not been associated with primary health care initiatives. Telehealth and technological advances may, however, help to decentralize audiological services to reach more people who have been unable to access hearing health care due to socioeconomic or societal barriers.

Examples of such decentralization include a pilot project in South Africa where community health care workers in severely underserved communities are using smartphones to conduct health registrations in people's homes. On their smartphones, a recently developed application (Swanepoel et al., 2014) is also installed and calibrated so that every household member receives a hearing screening. Noise levels are monitored and results uploaded to a centralized cloud-based server. Referrals are made for diagnostic testing at the local primary health care clinic. Usually, access to ear and hearing health services would require travel to distant hospital-based centers at significant travel costs and time with several visits back and forth likely. In an effort to decentralize basic ear and hearing health services, a teleaudiology clinic was established. Trained facilitators can manage the primary health care teleaudiology clinic, which provides automated testing with a diagnostic air and bone conduction audiometer that incorporates real-time noise monitoring and double attenuation (insert earphones covered by circumaural earphones) to allow for testing outside a soundbooth (Maclennan-Smith et al., 2013; Swanepoel, Mngemane, 2010). Results are automatically uploaded through a cellular network to a secure server from where a remote audiologist can make the necessary interpretation and recommendations to be sent back to the clinic. In addition to hearing assessment, video-otoscopy has been piloted to provide a remote diagnosis on ear disease by an otologist (Biagio, Swanepoel, Adeyemo, Hall, & Vinck, 2013; Biagio, Swanepoel, Laurent, & Lundberg, 2014). Based on these findings, limited medical treatment can be initiated at the clinic if recommended for audiological intervention. Patients can be referred directly for hearing aid fittings with their audiogram in hand.

This brings us to another example of decentralized audiological services in the form of hearing aid fitting, verification, support, and troubleshooting using telehealth. Validation reports have demonstrated the feasibility of these teleaudiology applications, and in some cases, these have already been included in clinical service delivery models (Campos & Ferrari, 2012; Ferrari & Bernardez-Braga, 2009; Pearce, Ching, & Dillon, 2009; Penteado et al., 2012; Poles & Ferrari, 2014). In addition, there has been increasing interest in extending these services to cochlear implant mapping and troubleshooting through telehealth (Eikelboom, Jayakody, Swanepoel, Chang, & Atlas, 2014; Hughes et al., 2012; McElveen et al., 2010; Ramos et al., 2009). These applications are sure to become more common and mobile into the future as a way to ensure easier access but also more convenience for patients.

Future Challenges for Teleaudiology

Whether we like it or not, teleaudiology will be part of ear and hearing health care services in the future. The challenge for audiologists will be to ensure that they lead the development of new service delivery models and the incorporation of new technologies to provide greater access and efficiency for patients with disabling hearing loss. Audiologists are the hearing health care specialists best qualified to ensure patients with hearing loss receive optimal care. Although audiologists may be hesitant to adopt new services that differ from existing clinical encounters, the danger is that in so doing, they abdicate the responsibility to champion and direct best practices in teleaudiology (Swanepoel, 2014).

Audiologists should welcome new technologies that could facilitate teleaudiology services once they are clinically validated and cost-efficiency benefits demonstrated. In the broader field of hearing health care delivery, there has been a recent development, sometimes wrongly associated with telehealth, which is the direct acquisition of hearing aids over the Internet. Internet hearing aid sales, however, are not a telehealth service, since there is no health professional taking responsibility for the patient as is required in a telehealth service delivery model. With the proliferation of Internet and mobile phone–based services, it is up to audiologists to consistently promote best practices. Telehealth services may utilize the Internet, but the audiologist remains accountable for the service provided. The profession of audiology should not shun new developments incorporating information and communication technologies but instead should lead the way to evaluate these for best outcomes in access and patient care (Swanepoel, 2014).

As teleaudiology services are validated, it is expected that these will become integrated components of existing ear and hearing health care service delivery models. This, however, brings up another major challenge to the uptake of teleaudiology—reimbursement for these services. Reimbursement and insurance coverage for telehealth is one of the most important barriers that have restricted its adoption to date (Bashshur, Shannon, Krupinski, & Grigsby, 2013). Where these services are not sufficiently reimbursed, teleaudiology will remain a promising but underutilized methodology for extending audiology services. On a legislative and regulatory level, much work remains to be done to find compatible ways in which these aspects can be accommodated while ensuring best practice service delivery (Swanepoel, 2014).

Summary

Audiology has always been a profession that has relied heavily on technology to diagnose and treat patients with hearing loss. As technologies change and advance more rapidly than ever before, audiological practices are bound to evolve. Teleaudiology is an evolution in hearing health care that is expanding access to care. As with all clinical professions, these models must be grounded firmly on research and evidence, ensuring best practices for the patients we serve.

What exactly the future of teleaudiology will look like is difficult to predict. There are important drivers that will direct what shape these services may ultimately take, but the particulars are impossible to foresee. The mobile and connectivity revolutions will no doubt mean that hearing health care will become more mobile and accessible. Traditional clinic-based services are likely to be supplemented by a more decentralized approach to increase access to care. As hearing loss increases with the aging world population, these developments may facilitate greater reach and impact for audiology at community-based levels. Whatever the future may hold, it is up to the audiology profession to harness the benefits of teleaudiology toward maximizing the reach and impact of limited audiological resources.

References

ABI Research. (2013). *45 million Windows phones and 20 million Black-Berry 10 smartphones in active use at year-end; enough to keep developers interested.* Retrieved January 30, 2014, from https://www.abi research.com/press/45-million-windows-phone-and-20-million-blackberry

Bashshur, R. L., Shannon, G., Krupinski, E. A., & Grigsby, J. (2013). Sustaining and realizing the promise of telemedicine. *Telemedicine and e-Health, 19*(5), 339–345.

Biagio, L., Swanepoel, D., Adeyemo, A., Hall, J. W., III, & Vinck, B. (2013). Asynchronous video-otoscopy by a telehealth facilitator. *Telemedicine and e-Health, 19*(4), 252–258.

Biagio, L., Swanepoel, D., Laurent, C., & Lundberg, T. (2014). Video-otoscopy recordings for diagnosis of childhood ear disease using telehealth at primary health care level. *Journal of Telemedicine and Telecare, 20,* 300–306.

Campos, P. D., & Ferrari, D. V. J. (2012). Teleaudiology: Evaluation of teleconsultation efficacy for hearing aid fitting. *Journal da Sociedade Brasileira de Fonoaudiologia, 24*(4), 301-308.

Clark, J. L., & Swanepoel, D. W. (2014). Technology for hearing loss—as we know it and as we dream it. *Disability and Rehabilitative Assistive Technology, 9,* 408–413.

Eikelboom, R. H., Jayakody, D., Swanepoel, D., Chang, S., & Atlas, M. D. (2014). Validation of remote mapping of cochlear implants. *Journal of Telemedicine and Telecare, 20,* 171–177.

Fagan, J. J., & Jacobs, M. (2009). Survey of ENT services in Africa: Need for a comprehensive intervention. *Global Health Action, 2,* 1–8.

Fatehi, F., & Wootton, R. (2012). Telemedicine, telehealth or e-health? A bibliometric analysis of the trends in the use of these terms. *Journal of Telemedicine and Telecare, 18*(8), 460–464.

Ferrari, D. V., & Bernardez-Braga, G. R. (2009). Remote probe microphone measurement to verify hearing aid performance. *Journal of Telemedicine and Telecare, 15,* 122–124.

Fiordelli, M., Diviani, N., & Schulz, P. J. (2013). Mapping mHealth research: A decade of evolution. *Journal of Medical Internet Research, 15*(5), e95.

Foulad, A., Bui, P., & Djalilian, H. (2013). Automated audiometry using Apple iOS-based application technology. *Otolaryngology-Head and Neck Surgery, 149,* 700–706.

Goulios, H., & Patuzzi, R. B. (2008). Audiology education and practice from an international perspective. *International Journal of Audiology, 47,* 647–664.

Handzel, O., Ben-Ari, O., Damian, D., Priel, M. M., Cohen, J., & Himmelfarb, M. (2013). Smartphone-based hearing test as an aid in the initial evaluation of unilateral sudden sensorineural hearing loss. *Audiology & Neurootology, 18*(4), 201–207.

Hughes, M. L., Goehring, J. L., Baudhuin, J. L., Diaz, G. R., Sanford, T., Harpster, R., & Valente, D. L. (2012). Use of telehealth for research and clinical measures in cochlear implant recipients: A validation study. *Journal of Speech, Language, and Hearing Research, 55*(4), 1112–1127.

Kelly, T., & Minges, M. (2012). Executive Summary. In T. Kelly & M. Minges (Eds.), *Information and communication for development 2012* (p. 3). Washington, DC: World Bank.

Khoza-Shangase, K., & Kassner, L. (2013). Automated screening audiometry in the digital age: Exploring uhear™ and its use in a resource-stricken developing country. *International Journal of Technological Assess to Health Care, 29*(1), 42–47.

Maclennan-Smith, F., Swanepoel, D., & Hall, J. W., III. (2013). Validity of diagnostic pure-tone audiometry without a sound-treated environment in older adults. *International Journal of Audiology, 52,* 66–73.

Mahomed, F., Swanepoel, D., Eikelboom, R. H., & Soer, M. (2013). Validity of automated threshold audiometry: A systematic review and meta-analysis. *Ear and Hearing, 34*(6), 745–752.

Margolis, R. H., Glasberg, B. R., Creeke, S., & Moore, B. C. (2010). AMTAS: Automated Method for Testing Auditory Sensitivity: Validation studies. *International Journal of Audiology, 49*(3), 185–194.

Margolis, R. H., & Morgan, D. E. (2008). Automated pure-tone audiometry: An analysis of capacity, need, and benefit. *American Journal of Audiology, 17,* 109–113.

McElveen, J. T., Blackburn, E. L., Green, J. D., McLear, P. W., Thimsen, D. J., & Wilson, B. S. (2010). Remote programming of cochlear implants: A telecommunications model. *Otology & Neurotology, 31,* 1035–1040.

Mester, A. F., & Stephens, S. D. G. (1984). Development of the audiometer and audiometry. *Audiology, 23*, 206–214.

Minges, M. (2012). *Key trends in the development of the mobile sector.* Washington, DC: International Bank for Reconstruction and Development/The World Bank. Retrieved January 30, 2014, from http://siteresources.worldbank.org/EXTINFORMATIONANDCOMMUNICATIONANDTECHNOLOGIES/Resources/IC4D-2012-Report.pdf

Pearce, W., Ching, T. Y. C., & Dillon, H. (2009). A pilot investigation into the provision of hearing services using teleaudiology to remote areas. *Australian and New Zealand Journal of Audiology, 31*(2), 96–100.

Penteado, S. P., de Lima Ramos, S., Battistella, L. R., Marone, S. A. M., Bento, R. F. (2012). Remote hearing aid fitting: Teleaudiology in the context of Brazilian public policy. *International Archives of Otorhinolaryngology, 16*(3), 371–381.

Poles, T. T., & Ferrari, D. V. (2014). Teleaudiology: Professional-patient communication in hearing aid programming and fitting via teleconsultation. *Audiology Communication Research, 19*(3), 299–309.

Ramos, A., Rodríguez, C., Martinez-Beneyto, P., Perez, D., Gault, A., Falcon, J. C., & Boyle, P. (2009). Use of telemedicine in the remote programming of cochlear implants. *Acta Oto-Laryngologica, 129*, 533–540.

Swanepoel, D. (2014). Tele-audiology. In J. Katz, M. Chaslin, K. English, L. J. Hood, & K. L. Tillery (Eds.), *Handbook of clinical audiology* (7th ed.). Alphen aan den Rijn, the Netherlands: Wolters Kluwer.

Swanepoel, D., Clark, J., Koekemoer, D., Hall, J., Krumm, M., Ferrari, D., . . . Barajas, J. J. (2010). Telehealth in audiology: The need and potential to reach underserved communities. *International Journal of Audiology, 49*, 195–202.

Swanepoel, D., Eikelboom, R., Hunter, M. L., Friedland, P. L., & Atlas, M. D. (2013). Self-reported hearing loss in baby boomers from the Busselton healthy aging study—Audiometric correspondence and predictive value. *Journal of the American Academy of Audiology, 24*(6), 514–521.

Swanepoel, D., Maclennan-Smith, F., & Hall, J. W. (2013). Diagnostic pure-tone audiometry in schools: Mobile testing without a sound-treated environment. *Journal of the American Academy of Audiology, 24*(6), 514–521.

Swanepoel, D., Mngemane, S., Molemong, S., Mkwanazi, H., & Tutshini, S. (2010). Hearing assessment—reliability, accuracy and efficiency of automated audiometry. *Telemedicine and e-Health, 16*(5), 557–563.

Swanepoel, D., Myburgh, H. C., Howe, D., Mahomed, F., & Eikelboom, R. H. (2014). Smartphone hearing screening with integrated quality control and data management. *International Journal of Audiology*, *53*, 841–849.

Swanepoel, D., Olusanya, B. O., & Mars, M. (2010). Hearing health-care delivery in sub-Saharan Africa—A role for teleaudiology. *Journal of Telemedicine and Telecare, 16*, 53–56.

Transactions of the American Otological Society. (1922, May). Fifth Annual Meeting, Washington, DC.

Windmill, I. M., & Freeman, B. A. (2013). Demand for audiology services: 30-Yr projections and impact on academic programs. *Journal of the American Academy of Audiology, 24*, 407–416.

World Health Organization. (2006). *Primary ear and hearing care training manuals.* Geneva, Switzerland: Author. Retrieved June 11, 2009, from http://www.who.int/pbd/deafness/activities/hearing_care/en/index.html

World Health Organization. (2008). *The global burden of disease: 2004 update.* Retrieved October 6, 2014, from http://www.who.int/healthinfo/global_burden_disease/2004_report_update/en/

World Health Organization. (2010). *Telemedicine: Opportunities and developments in member states, Volume 2.* Retrieved September 17, 2013, from http://www.who.int/goe/publications/goe_telemedicine_2010.pdf

World Health Organization. (2011). *Mortality data.* Geneva, Switzerland: Author. Retrieved from http://www.who.int/healthinfo/statistics/mortality/en/

World Health Organization. (2013a). *Millions of people in the world have a hearing loss that can be treated or prevented.* Retrieved September 13, 2013, from http://www.who.int/pbd/deafness/news/Millionslivewithhearingloss.pdf

World Health Organization. (2013b). *Multi-country assessment of national capacity to provide hearing care.* Geneva, Switzerland: Author. Retrieved March 6, 2014, from http://0-www.who.int.innopac.up.ac.za/pbd/publications/WHOReportHearingCare_Englishweb.pdf

Appendix A

Participant Survey: eLearning Courses

This questionnaire has been developed to provide Hear and Say with feedback on the Hear and Say WorldWide eLearning program. Information from this survey will enable us to identify ways to enhance the design and delivery of our courses in the future, as we endeavor to meet the needs of professionals worldwide.

Indicate which courses/seminars you enrolled in during 20 . . .

☐ Foundations of the Auditory-Verbal Approach

☐ Advanced Skills in Auditory-Verbal Practice

☐ Extension of Skills in AV Practice and Translational Research

☐ Other _____

Indicate your eLearning experiences prior to enrollment in the above course(s):

☐ Participated in eLearning courses as a learner

☐ Participated in eLearning courses as a teacher/lecturer

☐ Not previously participated in eLearning courses

Indicate your eLearning preferences for the next time you enroll in Hear and Say WorldWide courses/seminars:

☐ All courses delivered in the physical face-to-face mode

☐ All courses delivered in the blended cyber mode

☐ All courses delivered in the cyber face-to-face mode

Rate your level of interest in continuing to participate in the Hear and Say eLearning courses/seminars:

☐ High

☐ Medium

☐ Low

☐ None

Indicate areas where you would benefit from further training:

☐ Further develop my technical skills for accessing eLearning courses

☐ Increase my engagement with the asynchronous and synchronous features of the eLearning courses

☐ Both of the above

☐ No further training required at this time

Please comment:

_____

_____

Rate the ease of access to the asynchronous course materials on the Hear and Say dedicated platform:

☐ High

☐ Satisfactory

☐ Low

☐ Difficult

Please comment:

_____

_____

Rate the design of the asynchronous course content on the Hear and Say platform:

☐ Highly learner-friendly

☐ Moderately learner-friendly

☐ Not learner-friendly

☐ Other

Please comment:

_____

_____

Rate the quality and relevance of the course content:

☐ High

☐ Medium

☐ Low

☐ Other

Please comment:

_____

_____

Rate the ease of access to the cyber synchronous features on the Hear and Say platform:

☐ High

☐ Medium

☐ Low

☐ Other

Please comment:

_____

_____

Rate the weekly cyber synchronous (tutorial) sessions as

☐ Highly valuable

☐ Moderately valuable

☐ Less than valuable

☐ Of no value

Please comment:

_____

_____

In general, what is your opinion of the audio (VoIP) quality during the cyber synchronous (tutorial) sessions?

☐ Excellent

☐ Good

☐ Fair

☐ Poor

Please comment:

_____

_____

When the audio (VoIP) quality is less than optimal, what strategies have you found useful to manage this?
(For example, how do you manage when there is a delay in the audio? Are any specific troubleshooting strategies useful?)

Please comment:

Possible Problems	Useful Strategies
Delay in audio	
Echo/static/intermittent sound	
Cannot hear at all	
Other	

Rate the video (webcam) quality during the cyber synchronous (tutorial) sessions:

☐ Excellent

☐ Good

☐ Fair

☐ Poor

Please comment:

_____

_____

When the video (webcam) quality is less than optimal, what strategies have you found useful to manage this?
(For example, how do you manage when the video image is pixelated/fuzzy? Are any specific troubleshooting strategies useful?)

Please comment:

Possible Problems	Useful Strategies
Pixelated/fuzzy image	
Delay in video	
Drop out	
Cannot see lecturer/others at all	
Other	

Overall, how comfortable are you when participating in the cyber synchronous (tutorial) sessions?

☐ As comfortable as I would be if the sessions were face-to-face

☐ Comfortable

☐ Uncomfortable

☐ Very uncomfortable

Please comment:

_____

_____

How satisfied are you with the level of interaction/rapport you have with your lecturer and other participants online?

☐ As satisfied as I would be if the sessions were face-to-face

☐ Satisfied

☐ Dissatisfied

☐ Very dissatisfied

Please comment:

_____

_____

Rate your interest in continuing to participate in cyber synchronous sessions in future courses:

☐ High

☐ Medium

☐ Low

☐ Other

Please comment:

_____

_____

Would you recommend the Hear and Say eLearning courses to others?

☐ Yes

☐ No

Additional comments and/or recommendations:

_____

_____

_____

We thank you most sincerely for your valuable input!

Index

Note: Page numbers in **bold** reference non-text material.

271